THE DIABETIC FOOT

Edited by John E. McDermott, MD
Providence Medical Center
Seattle, Washington

Contributors

John Bowker, MD
Stephen F. Conti, MD
Dennis Jannise, CPed
Mark Myerson, Jr, MD
G. James Sammarco, MD
Matthew Tomaino, MD

Series Editor

Glenn B. Pfeffer, MD

American Academy of Orthopaedic Surgeons
6300 North River Road
Rosemont, IL 60018
1-800-626-6726

American Academy of Orthopaedic Surgeons
THE DIABETIC FOOT

The American Academy of Orthopaedic Surgeons Monograph Series is dedicated to Wendy O. Schmidt, American Academy of Orthopaedic Surgeons senior medical editor, 1987-1991.

Library of Congress Cataloging-in-Publication Data

The Diabetic Foot/edited by
John E. McDermott, MD
Library of Congress Catalog Card Number 95-8511
ISBN 0-89203-119-0

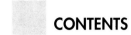

CONTENTS

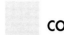 **CONTRIBUTORS**

John E. McDermott, MD
Providence Medical Center
Seattle, Washington

John Bowker, MD
Director, Foot and Ankle Services
Jackson Memorial Hospital
Department of Orthopaedics and Rehabilitation
University of Miami School of Medicine
Miami, Florida

Stephen F. Conti, MD
Assistant Professor
Chief, Division of Foot and Ankle Surgery
Department of Orthopaedic Surgery
University of Pittsburgh School of Medicine
Pittsburgh, Pennsylvania

Dennis Jannise, CPed
Medical College of Wisconsin
Milwaukee, Wisconsin

Mark Myerson, MD
Director, Foot and Ankle Services
The Union Memorial Hospital
Baltimore, Maryland

G. James Sammarco, MD
Volunteer Professor of Orthopaedics
Department of Orthopaedics
University of Cincinnati Medical Center
Cincinnati, Ohio

Matthew Tomaino, MD
Assistant Professor
Department of Orthopaedic Surgery
Division of Hand and Upper Extremity Surgery
Chief, Microvascular Surgery
University of Pittsburgh Medical Center
Pittsburgh, Pennsylvania

PREFACE

An umbrella of palm trees filters the equatorial sun as it enters the orthopaedic conference room through the tropical louvered windows. With its covered porticos and tall ceilings in its lush park setting, Singapore General Hospital speaks of Singapore's colonial period. The giant mahogany conference table with its oriental motif is an image from Somerset Maugham or James Michener, a setting that recalls the residency days lectures by Donald Qualls on "yaws and madura foot," orthopaedic foot challenges from the early 20th century. In his white tunic, Professor Balachandran completes the illusion, which is only broken by his comment, "it's all changed!"

Not only in modern urban Singapore but in the surrounding tropics and throughout the world, foot problems have changed. As the 20th century closes, from Miami to Seattle to Singapore, diabetes is now the significant disease of the foot and the leading cause of amputation.

In 1940 Joslin's classic study of the Navajo Indians of Arizona revealed only four cases of diabetes.[1] Twenty years later, 1% of the Navajo were diagnosed with diabetes,[2] and by the 1970s, 11% were diabetic and their complications accounted for 66% of lower extremity amputations carried out by the Indian Health Service.[2] Now diabetes represents 6% penetration in our populations and is a leading cause of hospitalization in modern America; it has penetrated other societies to an even greater extent.

The Committee on the Foot of the American Academy of Orthopaedic Surgeons, in cooperation with the American Orthopaedic Foot and Ankle Society, has long tried to communicate the significance of this problem. It is an honor to present this monograph, which outlines the current diagnosis and treatment strategies, as envisioned by leading surgeons of these two organizations. Our intention is to present a representative treatment protocol based on the successful team approach developed in multidisciplinary clinics. In presenting such a protocol, despite an effort to be inclusive, we have undoubtedly missed other successful concepts.

This monograph is the work of the contributors Mark Myerson, MD, "Amputation Surgery" and "Diabetic Neuroarthropathy," James Sammarco, MD and Stephen Conti, MD, "Infections," and Matthew Tomaino, MD "Soft-Tissue Reconstructive Surgery." Without their input, this effort would be in vain. I am also grateful to others who have contributed so much to the concepts of diabetic foot care, most notably William Wagner, MD, Richard Jacobs, MD, John Gould, MD, and Roger Mann, MD, and for the encouragement of John Bowker, MD, James Heckman, MD, and Michael Coughlin, MD. The editors and I also are indebted to Dennis Jannise, CPed, and Linda Hanna, LPN, CPed, for their input with respect to shoe wear management and patient education.

Acknowledgment must also be made to those who directly contributed to this publication: my co-authors' staffs; Shing Wai Yung, MD, who assisted with the bibliography; Sherrie Hess of my office; Molly Malone of Seattle Medical Steno, Inc; and, in particular, Jane Baque, the Academy's associate senior editor, who copyedited the manuscript.

It is proper also to acknowledge one's family. In my case, the text was dictated on family weekends and holidays, thus forcing my children to listen to their music via stereo earphones, but always smiling, I think, in support!

Joнn E. McDermott, MD

DEMOGRAPHICS

Despite advances in recognition and treatment, diabetic foot ulcers remain one of the most challenging skin problems faced by orthopaedic surgeons and other health care professionals.[3,4] Throughout the world, the diabetic foot is the leading cause of amputation. Currently, studies in the United States have shown that between 5% and 10% of all diabetics will require amputation, the rate increasing with age and showing some mild predilection for males, with a higher incidence among several ethnic groups.

Diabetic osteoarthropathy, the Charcot foot, is one of the most difficult fractures to manage. For the patient, it is a disabling problem, a fracture without "cause," frequently leading to poor results with severely impaired gait. For the physician, its frequently occult nature and dismal prognosis are a source of frustration. Unfortunately, the misunderstanding of this problem, on occasion, is even a cause of inappropriate litigious action.

Diabetic foot disease is progressive, with about half the patients facing a second amputation (the opposite foot) within 3 years.[5] The results of recent studies, however, have suggested that the incidence of diabetic foot disease, particularly the second amputation, can be improved through better preventative treatment.[6]

The westernization of Asia has resulted in an epidemic-like increase of diabetes in that region, mimicking that seen among the American Indian in the earlier part of the 20th century. In Singapore, with more than 30 McDonalds® restaurants among the hundreds of western restaurants, 15% of the mixed Chinese, Indian, and Malaysian population are diabetic. It is the sixth leading cause of death and the leading cause of amputation.[7] In contrast, Hong Kong, with a more traditional oriental diet, has seen an increase to only 1% of deaths.[8] In the United States, the amputation rate among American Indians is two to three times higher than that found in the general population.[9] Within this subgroup, the incidence of the disease itself is up to 50% greater. Changing of traditional diet, with substantially higher levels of carbohydrates, has been implicated in this phenomenon. A

"thrifty gene theory" has been proposed, whereby humans have the ability to store excess carbohydrate during times of plenty. When unchecked by periods of famine, the excessive carbohydrate consumption can overwhelm a previously less challenged genetic makeup.[9]

Atherosclerosis also plays an important role in the disease process of diabetes in the United States. The increasing degree of atherosclerotic change—the result of a higher incidence of atherosclerosis—is changing the clinical pattern of diabetes. The old concept that large-vessel disease is due to atherosclerosis and small-vessel disease is attributable to diabetes has now changed in the United States. Diabetes is becoming more commonly recognized as a combined disease, particularly in patients with type II, adult-onset diabetes. Thus, combined large- and small-vessel disease is now being seen with increasing frequency throughout the world as other populations turn to cholesterol-rich, high carbohydrate diets. As a result, surgical correction of large-vessel problems associated with diabetes has become increasingly necessary. Recently, the combination of large-vessel bypass in conjunction with distal revascularization procedures has been found to be successful for some of these combined disease problems.

The frequency of diabetes also results in other disease associations. While rare, the combination of diabetic neuropathy with other neurologic disease creates unusual and often insurmountable challenges. In the United States, the combination of diabetic neuropathy with stroke, Parkinson's disease, Charcot-Marie-Tooth disease, or Alzheimer's disease creates challenges to the control and treatment of both diseases. In tropical areas, the combination of diabetes with Hansen's disease results in rapidly disabling grotesque deformities (Fig. 1).[10]

The term "diabetes" was coined in the First century by Aretaeus, who described a "melting of flesh and limbs to urine," a reference to the polydipsia and polyuria that characterize this disease.[11] In the Fifth century, Susruta recognized the sweetness of the urine, but it was not until the 18th century that Dobson identified sugar in the urine. Modern treatment had its beginnings in 1921, when Banting and Best identified pancreatic extract as a prevention of the disease in a pancreatectomized dog. In sub-

FIGURE 1
Charcot changes. **Left,** Marked destruction of both osseus and soft-tissue elements with skin loss. **Right,** Radiographs show both Charcot changes in ankle and midfoot from combined disease, distal absorption typical of Hansen's change.

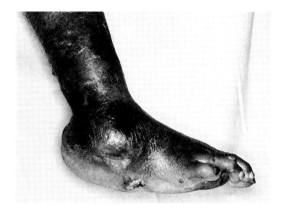
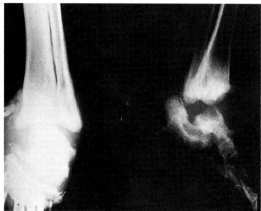

sequent research, however, diabetes was shown to be a far more complex problem than the mere lack of appropriate insulin levels in "glucose metabolism."

The hormone insulin is synthesized in the islets of Langerhans and is secreted in response to glucose levels. This response is dependent on both the presence of and function of the specialized islet cells. Although heredity was long recognized as a major factor in the pathologic process, recognition of the late acute onset of diabetes in only one of identical twins has given rise to the concept that diabetes might have other etiologies.[12] The onset of diabetes following a disease of possibly viral origin is now suspected.[13] On occasion, physical stress, infection, trauma, and surgery seem to aggravate the process. Hyperthyroidism, alteration in adrenocorticosteroids, and the hormonal changes during pregnancy have long been associated with alteration of glucose metabolism.

The common segregation of diabetes into type I, type II, or juvenile-onset versus adult is not physiologically based. However, such a classification is beneficial, particularly in predicting complications and in anticipating management difficulties. Type I (childhood onset) diabetes is more brittle; that is, changes in the blood sugar are more acutely influenced by insulin. Type II diabetes is often related to diet and obesity, has gradual onset in later life, and in the early stages can often be controlled with oral glucosuric medicines.

Diabetic neuropathy, the loss of myelinated and unmyelinated nerve fibers in diabetes, is thought to be a result of both vascular and metabolic factors. Ischemia at the microvascular level secondary to basement membrane change in small arterioles has been implicated. In addition, nerve biopsy studies suggest that the peripheral nerves are particularly sensitive to hyperglycemia and that this disturbed metabolism in nerve cells is responsible for their destruction. Neither of these concepts, however, apparently explains the lack of correlation between the degree of neuropathy and the degree of diabetes, particularly the not uncommon presentation of Charcot foot, before the metabolic problem is diagnosed or neuropathy recognized. Therefore, it is likely that a combination of these and perhaps other factors produce the nerve injury.[14]

 EPIDEMIOLOGY

The Diabetes Control and Complications Trial Research Group in 1993 published a study of

1,444 patients followed for 6.5 years to assess the progression of retinopathy, nephropathy, and neuropathy. Clinical neuropathy was defined as an abnormal neurologic examination consistent with peripheral neuropathy, plus either an abnormal nerve conduction in at least two peripheral nerves or unequivocal autonomic nerve testing. In this multicenter study, patients were randomly assigned to standard insulin control or to an intensive therapy administered either by external insulin pump or by three or more daily injections of insulin, guided by frequent blood sugar monitoring.

The developments of neuropathy and nephropathy were each significantly reduced by this strict monitoring of insulin levels. In patients assigned to the intensive management group, the incidence of retinopathy was reduced by 76% versus patients receiving the usual twice-daily insulin injections. Equally impressive, a 69% reduction in onset of neuropathy was reported. The findings represent a 3% incidence of neuropathy in those with intensive insulin management versus a 10% development in those with the usual insulin management during this 5-year study. These results would support the theory that more stringent insulin management will reduce the onset and progression of neuropathy. However, the study did note that there was a two- to three-fold increase in severe hypoglycemic reactions, which required management in the strict control group. No fatalities and no serious complications were reported despite this complication.

This and other studies, including the Swedish Intervention Study, support the need for optimum insulin control in diabetic patients. A therapy regimen designed to achieve blood glucose values as close to a normal range as possible would seem to prevent the onset and progression of neuropathy. Thus, such monitoring should be part of optimum diabetic foot care.

Research suggests that oxygen may also be a factor in the development of neuropathy and is a major factor in ulcer healing.[15] Studies have demonstrated that oxygen is necessary for macrophage mobility in wound debridement and the ingrowth of granulation tissue during wound healing. The function of some tissue growth factors is oxygen dependent. Further, some antibiotics, principally the aminoglycosides, depend on oxygen for their function. Thus, as the role of oxygen has become better understood, quite naturally, interest has turned to testing oxygen levels as a factor in diagnosis.[16]

Therefore, it is generally advised that tighter control of blood sugar fluctuation and the maintenance of more normal glucose levels will delay the onset of peripheral neuropathy and the progression of diabetic foot problems. Attention to controlling diabetes, educating the patient with respect to complications in the diabetic foot, and avoiding secondary risk factors (such as alcohol, tobacco, obesity, and deconditioning) all have been advocated to prevent foot problems. What has been shown to be of most benefit is the management and follow-up of at-risk patients in multidisciplinary foot clinics.

FOOT CLINIC ORGANIZATION

The clinical benefits of focused limb salvage, "foot-at-risk," and other specialized diabetic foot clinics have been demonstrated in a number of studies.[17] Amputation rates have declined and subsequent need for amputation of the opposite foot has also been dramatically diminished. Hickey and associates from St. Michael's Hospital Foot Clinic, Milwaukee, Wisconsin, compared their populations with nonclinic patients needing hospitalization for diabetic problems. They reported that the frequency of hospitalization was 23% less in patients from the focused foot clinic and that when admitted, the length of stay was reduced by almost two thirds, down from 9.7 to 3.5 days.[18]

Reiber[19] analyzed 1980 hospital discharge data and found that foot pathology was the most common complication leading to hospitalization among American diabetics. Her study demonstrated that multidisciplinary team approaches to diabetes have resulted in statistically significant reductions of morbidity and cost. This extensive study recommended that, regardless of the care setting, diabetic foot care guidelines should be viewed by a provider as recommended minimum practice levels, but she acknowledges that though these minimums are acceptable, they "are not intended to set a ceiling on professional excellence."

Focused clinics are unique in two ways; first, the enthusiastic emphasis given to the problem and second, the varied expertise that is brought to the care. Success of such clinics probably depends on both of these factors.

Studies document that both primary and tertiary care providers not only fail to evaluate the diabetic patient's feet, but also that there is a poor follow-up, even with respect to evaluating vision.[20] Thus, the foot clinic must function not only as a consultation center but it must also supply ongoing treatment and general diabetic follow-up.[21]

WHO IS IN CHARGE?

The qualifications of the clinic director are probably less important than the dedication and enthusiasm with which this individual approaches these difficult patients. Many clinics have found that an enthusiastic dedicated nurse director is best for overseeing day-to-day operations. Although medical directors of the clinics are often orthopaedic surgeons, other medical specialists are represented, including endocrinologists, dermatologists, general surgeons, vascular surgeons, and general practitioners. The key element is leadership.[22]

THE NURSE'S ROLE

It is the nurse who most often provides day-to-day operation of the clinic. The nurse's clinical responsibility begins with the initial interview of each patient, during which the patient's history begins to be gathered. In most clinics, it is the nurse who is responsible for the basic nail and skin care of the diabetic foot.

Patient education is the backbone of prevention for the diabetic patient, and such education must be ongoing.[23] The nurse has a primary role in this task, although all of the patient's caregivers must take part in the teaching. Education should be a part of each patient visit, with such education tailored to each patient's individual needs. It must include information about foot care and hygiene, specific instruction concerning the nails, and recommendations with respect to shoe wear and sock wear. The American Orthopaedic Foot and Ankle Society and several specialty organizations publish recommendations and patient information material. These materials should be provided and explained to patients and their caregivers.

Evaluation of the patient
The patient is quizzed concerning their general diabetic management; insulin and blood sugar levels are discussed. Attention is then focused on the foot and the patient's own capability and understanding of foot care.

Examination of the shoes and foot
The foot is examined with the patient actively involved. The skin is inspected with deliberate emphasis on examining the skin between the toes. Caregivers are involved if the patient is unable to fully participate in complete inspection due to impaired vision or agility. The importance of daily inspection is stressed as this procedure is performed. The shoes are inspected both externally and internally and then shaken out to make sure there is nothing in them that might rub against the foot. A deliberate inspection of the socks is performed again with patient participation and, at this time, shoe and sock precautions are reinforced (Outlines 1 and 2).

Education of the patient
Education of the patient and the caregiver is then done on an individual basis, tailored by inquiring as to the patient's life-style, activities of daily living, problems, and special needs. At each visit the patient is then counseled with respect to hygiene, foot precautions, routine foot care, and any special problems, such as ulcer or nail care.

Education must be all-encompassing; a diabetic patient is subjected to misinformation and frequently offered attractive alternatives to appropriate scientific care. In an article entitled "Alternative Medicine: Potential Dangers for the Diabetic Foot," the authors note patients whose ulcers were directly caused by such efforts.[24]

The skin and nails and footwear are carefully evaluated at each visit by the nurse. Foot care is performed most commonly by the nurse but may be performed in some clinics by a physical therapist or physician's assistant. Calluses are sanded or trimmed. Nails are trimmed and, if indicated, deformed nails are removed.

The goals of pedicare and education are for the patient to understand the problem and work toward the prevention of future complications.

In the education of nurses for their role in the foot care clinic, Hanna stressed the "three Es" (*see* Box) as a focus of patient understanding (LG Hanna, LPN, CPed, personal communication).

OUTLINE 1
Sock precautions

No mended socks

Wash socks inside out

If possible, use seamless stockings *or wear stockings inside out*

100% cotton is preferable; *80/40 blends are acceptable*

Light color socks are preferred *so that exudate can be identified*

Change socks daily or *more frequently if drainage is present*

OUTLINE 2
Shoe precautions

Shoe should be of soft material: should *produce no pressure*

Elasticized closures should be avoided: *fit should assure no shear effect*

Shoes should be inspected daily for intrusions: *tack in the sole*

Shoes should be shaken out before application: *avoid foreign body injury*

THE ROLE OF THE PEDORTHIST

With the increasing number of technical programs, and new college-level programs, there are increasing numbers of board-certified pedorthists. These shoe wear specialists provide the needed technical expertise in shoe wear modification and conservative treatment by insole fabrication. In some clinics, this needed capability can also be provided by a podiatrist, physical therapist, orthotist, prosthetist, or trained physician's assistants. In the clinical setting, such individuals must be able to participate in evaluation and must have the technical expertise to perform shoe wear modification. They need knowledge of the materials and the ability to fabricate the multidensity insoles often required in this type of care.

PHYSICAL THERAPIST AND ORTHOTIST

In some clinics, diabetic skin and nail care is provided by physical therapists. In this setting, their role may be similar to that of the nurse, assuming managerial and educational responsibilities as well as the responsibilities of direct care. Physical therapists who are to provide foot care need specific training with respect to foot wear and often find it beneficial to work directly with a pedorthist or orthotist. The basic request for all is training in modification of shoe wear and cast technique, as well as experience in wound care.

Similarly, orthotists practicing in the foot clinic will need a special interest in, and knowledge of, shoe wear modification. They need the technical expertise to measure for and mold custom insoles and custom shoe wear, or explicitly refer the client to a shoe facility that can provide such expertise. The orthotist's chief role is to provide orthoses (braces) for Charcot change in the hind foot and ankle, and to work in concert with the prosthetist to providing care to those patients who have had amputations.

THE PHYSICIAN STAFF

The diabetic patient represents a neurologic and vascular challenge; therefore, specialists in these two fields are necessary to provide the team approach to treatment. Most patients will need vascular evaluation and neurologic evaluation, while ongoing treatment probably more commonly involves an orthopaedic surgeon, podiatrist, dermatologist, or other practitioner with a particular interest in the diabetic foot. Those providers should have the knowledge and experience not only to manage the skin lesions, but also to understand and manage the underlying skeletal deformities and systemic problems commonly associated with the diabetic foot.

SUPPORT SERVICES

It would be extremely difficult to operate a specialized focus clinic without the availability of social service support; for as the patient's self-care capability wanes, patients and their families are challenged by multifaceted problems. A social service expert is needed to assist these patients with arrangements for home care, and to offer options for handling the problems of daily living that are associated with diminished musculoskeletal function often coupled with impaired vision.

As in any other clinic, there is a dependence on ancillary support services, such as laboratory support to evaluate blood and bacteria culture specimens and radiologic services to monitor Charcot changes. Vascular evaluation facilities are routinely necessary and must be readily available. The clinic itself needs the capability of Doppler evaluation and chem stick analysis and should be able to obtain specimens for those tests not performed in the clinic itself. Transcutaneous oxygen determination ($TCPO_2$), if not available in the clinic, should be readily accessible to the patient as part of the ulcer management decision.

 ## THE CLINICAL EVALUATION

In practice, it is often the nurse who begins the interview with the patient; reviewing the patient's history, in particular how the patient's diabetes has been controlled. Particular attention is paid to foot and shoe-related problems. This review is followed by focussing on a physical evaluation. The lower limbs are examined and the skin is inspected, including the soles of the feet and between the toes. Sock and shoe wear are evaluated. During this process, the patient is educated about checking the skin to avoid injury, avoiding improper sock wear, shaking out the shoes before donning and immediately reporting any problems.

The foot evaluation of the diabetic patient requires special focus. The history must be probing; the physical examination, extensive with respect to the foot and encompassing with respect to the musculoskeletal system. The challenge of management and the seriousness of complications necessitate time-consuming evaluation. An evaluation sheet can help in recording such findings (Fig. 2).

HISTORY

In obtaining the patient's general medical history, information regarding the onset and management of diabetes and other associated diabetic problems should be obtained. Special attention needs to be directed toward the patient's visual acuity and musculoskeletal problems that could affect gait. Past medical problems (particularly those involving the lower limb), history of infection, presence and man-

agement of vascular disease, as well as medications and medication problems should be noted. The family history is particularly important because the onset and progression of diabetes in family members may provide insight into the patient's prognosis.

The social history can uncover other risk factors, such as smoking, alcohol, and substance abuse. Previous foot treatment and any diagnostic testing or other significant evaluations should be discussed.

Diabetes has been called "a disease of denial." Psychologists suggest that in some patients the degree of denial equals that of the alcoholic. Thus, the psychological aspect of the evaluation may give insight to the patient's probable compliance and, thus, influence clinical decision-making.

EXAMINATION

The appropriate evaluation of the diabetic foot patient is a "clothes off," not "shoes off," procedure. Even during follow-up visits, full visualization of the lower limbs is often needed, with particular attention given to the vascular supply of the lower limbs (skin changes, venous congestion, edema).

General Musculoskeletal Evaluation

This examination must include gait evaluation, remembering such problems as ulcers of the first metatarsal head are often associated with disturbance in the rotary component of toe-off. Deformities of the hip and disabilities about the knee may cause abnormal stresses to the foot; for example, increased lateral foot and fifth metatarsal stress from genu varum. Strength testing not only of ankle muscles, but of knee and hip as well, is essential, particularly in planning conservative efforts with footwear modifications.

Focused Foot Evaluation

The foot type is determined and recorded. The cavus foot commonly represents challenges at the metatarsals and heel and the pronated foot, at the midarch. The skin turgor is evaluated, as is the presence or absence of hair, the color and temperature of skin, and the status of the nails. Special attention is directed to previous

FIGURE 2
Evaluation sheet for recording findings during evaluation of the diabetic foot.

(Adapted with permission from the St. Michael Hospital, Milwaukee, WI.)

Shoe difficulty: _____
Patterns of shoe wear: _____
Past medical diagnoses:
_____ Diabetes   Onset _____
_____ Inflammatory Arthritis
_____ Vascular Disease
_____ Gout
_____ Smoking _____
_____ Alcohol _____
_____ Other _____
What are your expectations of this visit: _____

Referring doctor: _____
Height _____ Weight _____
Temp___ Pulse___ Resp___ B/P_____
Allergies: _____
Medications: _____
Past surgical procedures: _____

R   L

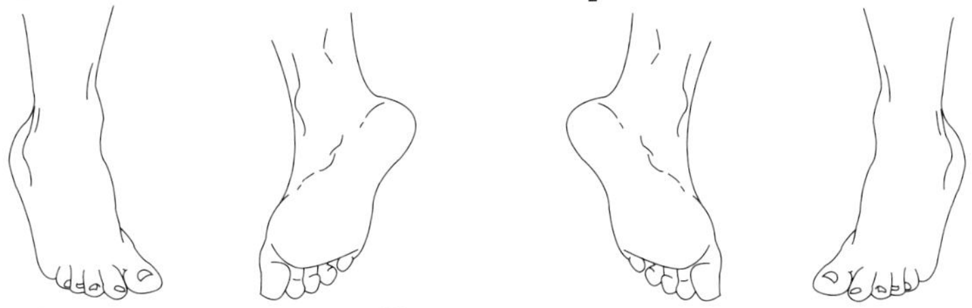

Pad deficient   PD
Tinels   T
Area of decreased sensation   °

pain   p   hard corn   hc
tender   x   soft corn   sc
verrucus v   end corn   ec
callus   c   warm   w
ulcer   u   scar   s

Neurovascular	R	L
Sensation		
Knee jerk		
Ankle jerk		
Pulses:		
Posterior Tibial		
Dorsalis Pedis		

Nails	R	L
	1 2 3 4 5	1 2 3 4 5
Ingrown		
Infected		
Incurvated		
Hypertrophic		
Onychomycosis		

Toes:	R	L
Hallux rigidus		
Hallux valgus		
Hallux pronation		
Eminence 1st MTP		
First MTP ROM		
First MTP spurs/ crepitus		
Hallux DIP ROM		
Hallux varus		
Bunionette		
Splaying		
Hammer		
Claw		
Mallet		
Overriding		
Neuroma		
Gait		

Ankle	R	L
ROM: DF		
ROM: PF		
Instability		
Hindfoot		
Standing position		
ROM: Inversion		
ROM: Eversion		
Single limb heel rise test		
Midfoot		
Standing position		
ROM: Pronation		
ROM: Supination		
Forefoot		
Standing position		
Supinated (Fixed/Mobile)		
Pronated (Fixed/Mobile)		

X-Ray

_____ Standing AP/Lateral foot
_____ With oblique
_____ Standing AP/Lateral ankle
_____ With mortise view
_____ Other _____

Findings:

Lab Orders _____ Uric acid _____ CBC _____ RA _____ Sed rate _____ Other _____
_____ Harris mat
_____ Photograph

Diagnosis:

Treatment:

_____ Pedicure program _____
_____ Pedorthics _____
_____ Orthotist _____
_____ Medication _____
_____ Surgery _____
_____ Return _____

_____
MD Signature

FIGURE 3
Neutral position. Neutral position is determined by the examiner palpating the medial border of the talus and rotating the foot from adduction to abduction. (Courtesy of R. Luke Bordelon, MD)

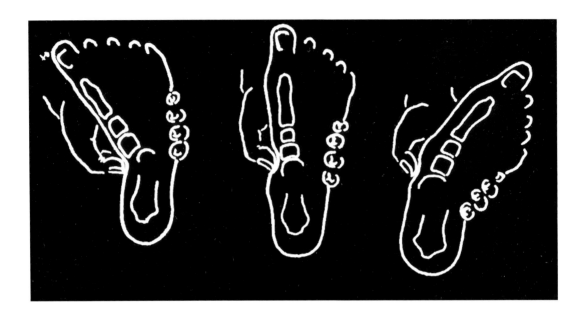

incisions, injuries, and deformities. The skin, including the areas between the toes, is examined for any evidence of breakdown, infection, or pressure.

Mobility is individually evaluated at all joints. Clawing of toes, rotational deformities, and bunion-related problems increase foot risk. The midfoot is palpated, and the examiner looks for any early signs of inflammation, especially swelling or increased warmth, which could herald Charcot change. The suppleness of the foot is determined by bringing the foot to a neutral position with respect to the talonavicular joint (Fig. 3). The range of motion of the forefoot in supination and pronation is then evaluated. Similarly, the "Block test," in which a block is placed under either the medial or lateral forefoot to elevate it, can also be used to determine the degree of midfoot pronation or supination.

Shoe Wear Evaluation

Patients and their caregivers cannot be expected to understand the seriousness of the shoe wear problem unless the provider shows a significant degree of concern. This includes taking the time to evaluate footwear at each visit. The patient's socks should be noted and at this time the patient is counseled regarding sock wear. The shoe wear is checked inside and out while routinely advising the patient to shake out the shoes and examine the inside of the shoes for problems each time they are put on. Shoes must be evaluated with respect to size, fit, condition (eg, signs of wear), and appropriateness; the uppers should be soft and the soles and heel abrasions shock absorbing. Proper fitting shoes should cause no areas of skin pressure or shear.

The Vascular Examination

The vascular examination begins proximally and progresses down to the dorsalis pedis and posterior tibial vessels. Pulse status, warmth, and color should be noted and documented on a flow sheet.

Classic studies have taught that Doppler-derived ankle/arm systolic pressure indices can be a predictor of success in the management of vascular and diabetic ulcers. Doppler ultrasound can be used to measure arterial flow patterns and to assess quantitative blockage of the arterial

FIGURE 4
Doppler laser. (Reproduced with permission from Brodsky JW: Outpatient diagnosis and care of the diabetic foot, in Heckman JD (ed): *Instructional Course* *Lectures 42*. Rosemont IL, American Academy of Orthopaedic Surgeons, 1993, pp. 121-139.)

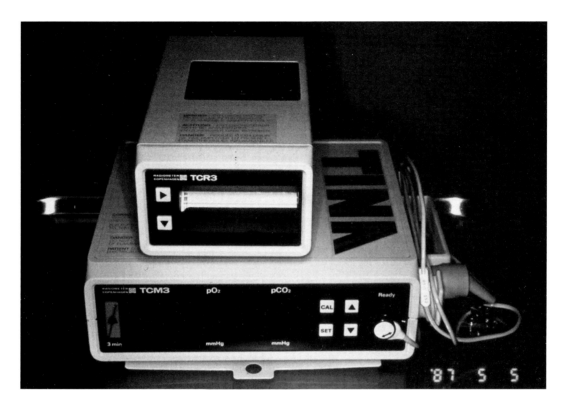

tree. Systolic pressures are obtained sequentially at various points along the leg, foot, and distally to the toes. Lower limb pressure is divided by the brachial artery pressure to calculate the ischemic index (Fig. 4). Ankle/arm indices and/or Doppler studies are performed on the initial visit and should be reported periodically, particularly with any change in foot status. However, Doppler ultrasound measures the status of the larger arteries and not the skin capillaries. Because capillaries are also important in healing, Doppler ultrasound may be unreliable in the presence of obstructed or calcified small vessels. However, recent studies have eroded some of the confidence once placed in this test. The ankle/arm pressure indices can be influenced by the degree of atherosclerosis and do not provide insight concerning distal arterial run-off. Use of a laser Doppler can be more accurate because the per-

fusion of the skin is determined.[25] Studied Doppler pressure evaluation is most appropriate for larger vessels. But standard Doppler and even laser Doppler give no insight into the amount of oxygen carried by the red blood cells or the tissue's ability to participate in the diffusion process. This can only be done by transcutaneous oximetry.

Although the accuracy provided by the Doppler ischemic index is usually satisfactory, in some patients with extensive peripheral vascular disease or medial sclerosis of the vessels, measurement of the Doppler index is impossible because the vessel walls cannot be compressed. If pulsatile flow is audible, the amputation level is better determined based on the overall skin condition, temperature, and presence or absence of infection. The classic determination of ankle/arm indices, with 0.45 being a guideline to tissue

FIGURE 5
Left, Transcutaneous oxygen probe measures oxygen defusion at skin surface. **Right,** Probe applied to anticipated level of amputation in a diabetic patient.

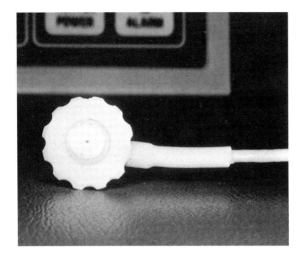
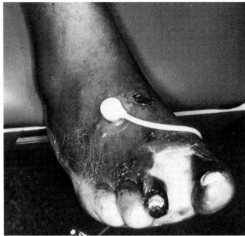

survival, has been widely questioned. in 1964 Carter demonstrated that the ankle/arm measure was abnormal in 80% of those with arterial disease. Studies performed on diabetics at the New Jersey Veterans' Administration Hospital have suggested such predictability of healing was accurate in only a third of the patients studied, while a determination of transcutaneous oxygen was 100% accurate in predicting both wound healing and determining appropriate amputation level in diabetic patients.[26]

The New Jersey Veterans' Administration Hospital analyzed the various techniques of vascular evaluation and found that the best predictor of wound healing or amputation success is $TCPO_2$ level. This measures the actual oxygen available to the tissue, which is the critical factor.

$TCPO_2$ determination is most commonly performed using the neonate monitoring device utilized in newborn nurseries (Fig. 5). The test is time-consuming, requiring 20 minutes to allow temperature stabilization of the probe. (Temperature stabilization is necessary to measure oxygen partial pressure in the skin tissue itself.) This test should not be confused with the "pulse oximeter," used during anesthesia, which indicates the degree of oxygenation in arterial blood. The $TCPO_2$ determination is the actual level of O_2 saturation measured as diffusion at the skin's surface.

Current technique calls for the measurement of $TCPO_2$ above the ankle and dorsum of the foot or other areas of concern, such as nonhealing wound sites. If the measurements fall below 30 mm Hg, wound healing is highly improbable; an ulcer will often fail to heal and skin flap and other surgery should not be contemplated. Normal values vary with individuals, but fall between 60 and 90 mm Hg, with levels between 30 and 40 mm Hg questionable with regard to wound healing.

$TCPO_2$ determination begins with the patient being evaluated, usually in at least four sites. Bilateral determination is done whenever necessary. The tests should be performed in a relatively warm room because this allows a base-level temperature to be achieved more rapidly prior to the determination by preventing vasoconstriction.

The small probe is placed on the area to be measured (the dorsum of the foot, for example). After a constant baseline body temperature has been reached, readings are taken in millimeters of mercury at 10, 20, and 30 minutes. The actual level is a product of the skin's vascular diffusion rate and of the patient's current oxygen saturation. As stated, a finding of less than 40 mm Hg should denote the possibility of delayed wound healing, values below 20 mm Hg will not support tissue healing and further breakdown is usually inevitable.

The measurement of pulse wave form and the determination of segmental pressures or toe pressures also provide good indications and are widely used.[27] Most authors agree, however, that the correlation is not as predictable as the actual determination of available oxygen to the tissue being measured.

Cutaneous temperature also can be correlated with skin blood flow using venous occlusion plethysmography. Many commercially available skin thermistors and thermocouples are accurate enough for determining the level of amputation (see *Amputation Surgery*).

If arterial insufficiency is present and bypass surgery is performed, amputation may be possible at a more distal level than would have been possible without revascularization. The status of the arterial circulation is the major determinant of wound healing and should be relied on in some way to assist in determining the level of amputation.

A high percentage of diabetic patients need arteriography for major vessel evaluations. However, arteriography only reflects the status of the larger arteries and not the arterioles and skin capillaries that are also important in healing. Furthermore, involvement of the major vessels is usually patchy; if these vessels are gradually occluded, a collateral blood supply develops, which may support an adequate peripheral circulation. Therefore, the absence of pulses in major limb vessels does not necessarily indicate severe ischemia. This has the same implications for arteriography and conservative amputations may still heal in spite of arteriographic occlusion.

The Neurologic Examination

Neurologic examination records motor strength, reflexes, and light touch and vibratory sensation determination.[28] Light touch sensation is best checked with the Semmes-Weinstein filaments (Fig. 6). The usual sensory wheel or pinprick test is inappropriate not only because of the risk of skin penetration in such infection-prone individuals, but also because it is not accurate enough for evaluation of diabetic neuropathy (Fig. 6). The Semmes-Weinstein filament

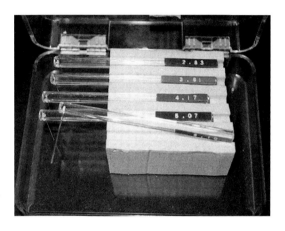

FIGURE 6
Semmes-Weinstein microfilaments. (Reproduced with permission from Brodsky JW: Outpatient diagnosis and care of the diabetic foot, in Heckman JD (ed): *Instructional Course Lectures 42.* Rosemont, IL, American Academy of Orthopaedic Surgeons, 1993, pp 121-139.)

technique should be performed at the initial evaluation, and a sensory "map" should be made. The map will document sensory deprivation levels based on the filaments used. Three filaments are commonly employed beginning with the 1 g. If sensation is not noted, the next larger filament is used, progressing through 10 g and 75 g. The filament rod is pressed to the skin until it bends. The procedure is repeated beginning distally with the toes, the midfoot, the hindfoot, the ankle, and the distal leg. The determination is best repeated at least two times per year or following any significant problem.

Recently, a multicenter study and expanded sensory evaluation has been developed for evaluation of the Charcot foot. The modified examination has been developed for computer study. It evaluates sensory, autonomic, and motor nerve function by history and specific sensory entry. This type of evaluation form serves as an adjunct to the usual sensory mapping evaluation sheets commonly found in foot care clinics.

Nutritional Evaluation

The diabetic patient's general metabolic and nutritional status should always be considered impaired. In the preoperative patient, the white blood cell (WBC) count, temperature, and fasting

TABLE 1
Risk criteria and recommended management

Risk Category	Problem	Recommendations
0	Diabetes Normal sensation +/− foot deformity	Yearly follow-up Normal footwear Footwear education
1	Diabetes Loss of sensation No deformity	6-month follow-up Soft insoles Patient education
2	Diabetes Loss of sensation Foot deformity	4-month follow-up Custom-molded foot orthosiss Prescribed footwear Patient education
3	Diabetes Loss of sensation Foot deformity History of ulceration	2-month follow-up Custom-molded foot orthosis Prescribed footwear Patient education

blood sugar are significantly correlated with surgical success or failure. The basal daily energy expenditure of a 70-kg male is approximately 1,800 kcal, but these energy requirements are increased by about 40% during severe infection and particularly surgery. Catabolic losses are worse during hospitalization. Severe nutritional depletion is indicated by an albumin concentration of less than 3.0 g/dl and a total lymphocyte count (% lymphocytes × WBC count) of less than 1,500 indicates immunosuppression. These patients all benefit from nutritional supplementation during hospitalization for infection.

FOLLOW-UP

The insidious nature of the diabetic problem, the common psychological denial process, coupled with the lack of pain, contribute to noncompliance on the part of the diabetic patient. These factors together with the occult nature of progression make the establishment of specific follow-up visits an essential part of clinic management.

In an effort to categorize patients with respect to frequency of treatment and determining appropriateness of follow-up management, risk criteria have evolved based on the evaluation. Recommended follow-up considers history, foot status, and sensory levels. St. Michael's Hospital Clinic, Milwaukee, Wisconsin, recommends routine 6-month follow-up evaluations for any diabetic patient with sensory deprivation. With foot deformities, the patient is evaluated more frequently; if there is history of ulceration, the patient is evaluated at least bimonthly (Table 1).

Following skin and nail care and any necessary treatment, the patient is given a specific date for a return appointment. At this time, the nurse verifies the patient's understanding of any self care instructions given by other clinic staff; ie, ulcer care, medication use, shoe modifications.

PATIENT EDUCATION

The nature of diabetes makes education a paramount activity of the treatment team. The success of the specialized clinic depends on the patient's own efforts with respect to prevention and participation in the healing process.

Each clinic visit, the nurse or other designated staff person spends time in individual patient education. At the initial evaluation, many clinics use a formal educational program. The Foot Clinic of St. Michael's Hospital, Milwaukee, Wisconsin, has developed a videotape for such purposes. Many of the hospital-based clinics use formal diabetic education classes with time devoted to the problems of the foot. These efforts, however, should be augmented by a one-on-one teaching effort by the clinic staff.

As with most educational efforts, the more focused and specific the education is to the patient's need, the more likely it is to be effective. All patients should be counseled as to foot precautions. A handout, such as is illustrated in Outlines 1 and 3, can be helpful. The patient is educated with respect to shoe selection and reminded repeatedly concerning the specifics of shoe- and foot-related diabetic problems (Outline 2).

The patient with a foot ulcer needs to be educated in how to care for the ulcer, with reminders concerning foot hygiene and, of course, continued effort with respect to prevention and shoe selection.

For the Charcot patient, education focuses on shoe selection, constant monitoring of swelling, careful daily evaluation of the opposite foot, and standard educational efforts about the foot.

Educational materials are available from many sources. One of the most widely available resources is a local chapter of the American Diabetes Association. Many such chapters will assist in actual patient education programs and would welcome the referral of a newly diagnosed patient to their organization, for such networking can be mutually beneficial to patient and clinic and focus group.

A frequently overlooked aspect of education is the patient's caregiver. The diabetic patient can be dependent on the caregiver, so that education of the caregiver is as important as that of the patient. It is the caregiver who often must carry out the actual recommendations of the management team, particularly as the patient progresses through the usual complications of both the musculoskeletal system and vision. This education process often must involve the social worker and home health care services provider because the specific caregiver may not be the one who attends the clinic with the patient.

DIABETIC NAIL CARE

The mainstay of the diabetic foot clinic is its nail care program. Diabetic hypertrophic nails associated with onychomycotic deformities are the most common causes of patient referral. The routine care of the nails along with skin care is an essential part of diabetic foot management. In most clinics, this routine work is performed by a nurse, physical therapist, or physician's assistant. Because of the risk of injury and infection, it must be skillfully done, which necessitates both demanding technique and the proper tools. In dealing with particularly diseased nails, the patients must be forewarned that spontaneous avulsion may take place and that infection can occur despite the most meticulous care.

TECHNIQUE

Prior to beginning nail care, health care providers must assure their own personal safety (Fig. 7). Goggles as well as an appropriate gown should be worn in addition to gloves. A mask and hair covering are advisable, particularly if power equipment is used. The decision to use a prep prior to pedicare is somewhat up to each individual. Certainly, if there is soiling or heavy contamination, a brief scrub is beneficial. Soaking, however, will tend to macerate the nail, making it difficult to cut and causing it to plug the sanding equipment.

EQUIPMENT

Basic equipment includes a selection of scissors, nail trimmers, file, hemostat, and perhaps a bone rongeur. In addition, if the nail needs to be split, an anvil-type nail splitter is far superior to the scissors (Fig. 7). Once mastered, however,

FIGURE 7
Pedicare equipment. Nail clippers, nail splitter, file, hemostat for debridement, electric drummel, eye protection, face mask, hair protection, and clothing cover.

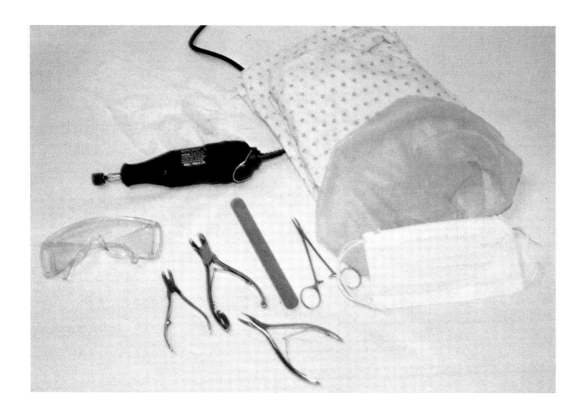

the most valuable piece of equipment is a hobby type hand-held rotary sanding device with a speed control. These are available at hardware stores and most hobby shops. Use of the rechargeable type avoids the inconvenience of cords and plugs. Small, disposable sanding cylinders that fit over a drum device facilitate easy between-patient changing (Fig. 7).

TECHNIQUE

Large hypertrophic nails can be first approached with either double-action rongeur or bone-cutter. Normal nails are power sanded or can be easily trimmed with a standard nail trimmer or scissors. The rough spurs and fragments are then sanded with the hobby-type hand-held sanding device or if not available, a hand sander. In using the hand-held sanding device, care must be taken to prevent tissue heating or injury. Skin can be protected by placing a small trimmed piece of exposed X-ray film beneath the nail (Fig. 8). A curette and hemostat can be used to remove debris from beneath the nail edge. If the nail has retained reasonable margin anatomy, care must be taken to trim the nails straight across to avoid the tendency to ingrow at the nail margin.

Callus formation, a leading cause of problems for the diabetic, can be managed in a similar fashion. A Podi or rounded #17 scalpel blade is preferred for sharp paring to avoid skin injury. With some experience, the hand-held sanding device also can be used for callus management.

FIGURE 8
Sanding technique, drummel is applied with minimum pressure, adjacent skin protected with a strip of X-ray film.

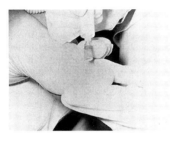 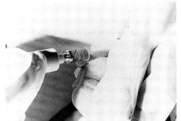 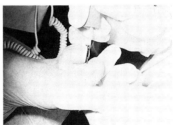

Again, great caution must be used to avoid heat buildup in thickened calluses particularly in patients lacking normal sensation.

Infected nails and ingrown nails require appropriate surgical management with debridement and, if indicated, matricectomy. Partial resections of the distal nail margin are to be condemned. In general, these will only temporarily relieve the impalement process and ultimately a second procedure, such as partial matricectomy, will be necessary and the patient subjected to further risk.

 MATRICECTOMY

A matricectomy may be either a "total" removal of the entire nail or subtotal excision, a "partial" excision of just the nail margin. In advanced nail disease, often simple nail removal will suffice with regrowth resulting in less deformity and some relative little recurrence. After a true matricectomy, however, no regrowth is anticipated because the nail growth plate is removed. If the nail is grossly deformed and is a constant threat to infection, a complete matricectomy is advised. However, for nail margin problems such as ingrown nails, the partial matricectomy will often suffice. In the face of infection, it is best that the nail plate not be disturbed, and regrowth anticipated.

In the neuropathic foot, anesthesia is rarely necessary; however, if required, a toe block is performed. A small additional injection of anesthetic at each skin corner and below the toe tip is often helpful. Following the usual preparation if a partial matricectomy is to be done, an Anvil-type nail splitter is used and the nail split from distal to proximal at the appropriate position (Fig. 9). A Freer elevator can then be used to lift the nail, which then is forcibly removed with the hemostat. In infected or ingrown nails, only necrotic and infected material is removed and an antibacterial dressing is applied.

If an obliterative matricectomy is to be performed, two small skin wedges are removed at the corners of the nail base. The nail matrix is then sharply dissected and removed by curettage from the distal phalanx dorsal surface. If the equipment is available, the nail matrix may be destroyed with laser technique. The tissue under the nail contains nail growth potential and this nailbed should be superficially debrided. The skin folds at the margin are excised along with the eponychium tissue at the nail base. A suture is then placed in each corner wedge to facilitate closure and hemostasis. A Xeroform® antibacterial or other nonadherent gauze is placed and a compressive dressing applied.

The patient is provided pain medication, if needed, and antibiotics, if appropriate. They are instructed to return in 3 to 4 days, at which time the dressing is removed and the patient is instructed on follow-up soaks. If infection has been present (ie, marginal resection for ingrown nail), the soaks are begun in the immediate postoperative period and preferably an earlier follow-up is scheduled.

FIGURE 9
Matricectomy technique. **Left,** Matricectomy instruments, minor surgery set-up plus nail splitter, rongeur, curette, and rubber band tourniquet. **Right,** Partial matricectomy. Relief incisions are placed at nail base angle and soft tissue and underlying nail bed are dissected. Anvil-type nail splitter application is used.

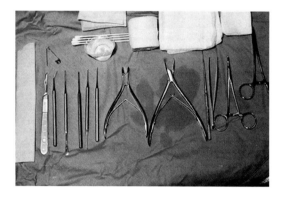
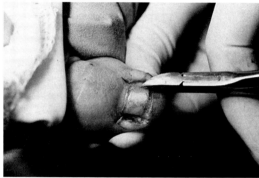

 ULCER MANAGEMENT

CLASSIFICATION

Foot and ankle diabetic ulcers (mal perforans) are classified in order to provide optional guidelines for treatment. The more refined the classification system, the more precisely a treatment protocol can be defined. Many classification systems have been proposed. Recently, Brodsky has proposed an elaborate ischemia classification system that lends itself to a refined treatment protocol[29] (Table 2). The earlier classification proposed by Wagner, however, is more widely accepted and is perhaps better understood.[30,31]

The Wagner classification describes lesions based on the depth of the wound. This approach is similar to that used for classifying burns. Superficial lesions represent grade I; full-thickness ulceration, grade II; ulcer penetrating into bone, grade III; and those ulcers complicated by gangrene, grades IV or V, depending on extent (Table 3).

During each office visit, the ulcer is examined and classified and its status with respect to the inflammatory response and infection is determined. First, all hypertrophic calluses are removed. The depth can then be determined by inspection. The ulcer is then measured and inspected. A piece of clear kitchen plastic is placed over the wound to prevent contamination of the chart recording. The wound is traced on a piece of clear X-ray film, which is dated and placed in the patient's chart (Fig. 10).[27] The changes in contour and size of the ulcer can then be accurately documented and compared at subsequent follow-up visits to determine treatment progress. The depth of the ulcer is ascertained by probing it with a sterile cotton-tipped applicator. The depth is also recorded. Only through such accurate delineation can the true success or failure of treatment be ascertained.

CONSERVATIVE TREATMENT

Debridement

For healing the diabetic ulcer needs to be debrided to a clean granulating "pink" skin margin and a granulating base. Because like all wounds the diabetic heals from a healthy skin margin, any hypertrophic callus, eschar, or hypertrophic basal granulation tissue tends to block this healing at the skin margins. Ulcers that are associated with a hypertrophic base and proliferative inflammatory response are best managed with wound-type treatment, such as

TABLE 2
The "depth/ischemia" classification of
diabetic foot lesions

Grade	Definition	Treatment
Depth Classification		
0	The "at risk" foot. Previous ulcer or neuropathy with deformity that may cause new ulceration	Patient education Regular examination Appropriate shoe wear and insoles
1	Superficial ulceration, not infected	External pressure relief: Total contact cast, walking brace, special shoe wear, etc
2	Deep ulceration exposing tendon or joint (with/without superficial infection)	Surgical debridement → wound care → pressure relief if closes and converts to grade 1 (PRN antibiotics)
3	Extensive ulceration with exposed bone and/or deep infection: ie, osteomyelitis, or abscess	Surgical debridements → ray or partial foot amputations → IV antibiotics → pressure relief if wound converts to grade 1
Ischemia Classification		
A	Not ischemic	Adequate vascularity for healing.
B	Ischemia without gangrene	Vascular evaluation (Doppler, $TCPO_2$, arteriogram, etc) → vascular reconstruction PRN.
C	Partial (forefoot) gangrene of foot	Vascular evaluation → vascular reconstruction (proximal and/or distal bypass or angioplasty) → partial foot amputation
D	Complete foot gangrene	Vascular evaluation → major extremity amputation (BKA, AKA) with possible proximal vascular reconstruction

(Reproduced with permission from Brodsky JW: The diabetic foot, in Mann RA, Coughlin MJ (eds): *Surgery of the Foot and Ankle*, ed. 6. St. Louis, MO, Mosby Year Book 1992, pp 1361-1467.)

wet-to-dry soaks. A variety of chemicals have been advocated and several commercially prepared wound treatment protocols exist; however, there is no real documentation that such agents represent any benefit over the simple wet-to-dry soaks.

Hypertrophic granulation tissue, small bits of necrotic wound debris, and superficial bacterial contamination are easily removed using wet-to-dry soak technique. An open-weave, gauze-type dressing such as Kerlix® is placed on the wound and then soaked. After the dressing dries, it is removed. The attachment of wound particulates to the dressing in the drying process facilitates on its removal a surface debridement of those elements adhering to the gauze.

The technique for a wet-to-dry soak is carried out in the following manner. The patient is instructed to place one layer gauze dressing on the wound and wrap the dressing to the foot with no more than two or three layers of a similar open-weave type gauze. (Restricting the depth of layers will facilitate more rapid drying, with less tissue maceration.) The patient then is

TABLE 3
Wagner classification and recommended management

Stage	Classification	Recommendations
0	Pressure area on foot aggravated by footwear	Footwear modification
I	Open but superficial ulceration	Local treatment Footwear modification
II	Full-thickness ulceration	Occlusive cast Footwear modification
III	Full-thickness ulceration with secondary infection	Debridement Antibiotics
IV	Infected area with local gangrene	Antibiotics Local amputation Hyperbaric O_2
V	Ulceration with extensive gangrene, foot and leg	Regional amputation Antibiotics Rehabilitation

FIGURE 10
An example of the chronologic record of ulcer healing made by tracing the ulcer outlines into the patient chart. (Reproduced with permission from Brodsky JW: Outpatient diagnosis and care of the diabetic foot, in Heckman JD (ed): *Instructional Course Lectures 42.* Rosemont, IL, American Academy of Orthopaedic Surgeons, 1993, pp 121-139.)

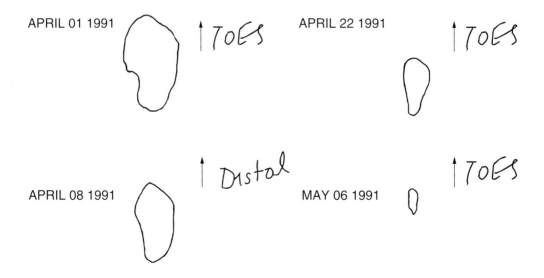

instructed to soak the foot and dressing in or with a solution of choice. (Normal saline or Burow's works as well as more exotic solutions and is cost-effective. Soap solutions are too drying, and peroxide should never be used.) After 10 to 20 minutes of soaking, the foot and dressing are allowed to air-dry usually a period of 30 minutes to 1 hour and the dressing is removed. This process is best repeated three to four times a day for active debridement and to enhance wound healing. In another simpler and equally effective method, the gauze in contact with the wound surface is moistened with normal saline and then wrapped with dry gauze. This is repeated two or three times daily. Maceration of tissue with any type of soaks must be avoided. Dry skin can be treated with lotion, balm, or vegetable shortening, such as Crisco®.

Ulcer Debridement at the Office Visit

Most foot ulcers involving particularly the plantar aspect of the foot will require active debridement at each office visit. Such debridement often can be accomplished bluntly using either a pickups or hemostat to separate and then peel eschar and hypertrophic callus from the area. Care is always taken to avoid skin tears in the asensory foot. It is often even possible to use a gloved fingernail to dissect between the dermis and the granulating eschar area—a most simple and safe means of dissection.

A small scalpel can then be used to trim any residual hypertrophic callus or eschar and dissect the usually white, necrotic ulcer margin. For tissue in-growth, this margin must be cleared of all nonviable tissue preferably without causing active bleeding. When the dissection is completed, the ulcer margins should be pink with "healthy" dermis margin capable of regeneration.

As noted, attention needs to be paid to the base of the ulcer itself. The presence of thickened hypertrophic granulation tissue from the base can mechanically block the ingrowth of skin from the dermal margins of the wound.

Dressings

The same basic principles apply to dressing the diabetic ulcer as apply to any other delicate skin lesions, such as burn wounds. There is little evidence that any substance except perhaps oxygen benefits the delicate physiologic in-growth of wound healing. Certainly, toxic paint-ing (iodine, etc) or the use of a tissue-destructive solution such as hydrogen peroxide should be avoided. Burn-type regimens have not worked as well in the diabetic ulcer as they have in burns. Newer physiologic-type dressings do seem to have some enhanced healing potential, and several centers have reported benefits from platelet-derived growth factors applied to the ulcer area.[32] While early reports have shown some promise, healing time is markedly slower than ambulatory treatments using casts or boots. At this time, application of growth-enhancement substances is still investigational (see *Wound Growth Factors*).

The more universally accepted approach seems to be that of a physiologic, burn-type dressing, such as DuoDerm® over the freshly debrided ulcer. The patient is instructed to remove the dressing after several days. Often, however, no dressing need be applied but rather the area bathed and covered with clean socks, which are to be changed several times a day to absorb exudate and to assist in the physiologic debridement process. This technique is always used in conjunction with a total-contact insole diabetic type footwear management. Initial ulcer management usually involves occlusive casting, and the cast is usually the dressing of choice. Subsequent healing can be accomplished in a carefully managed clinical follow-up setting with expertly fitted shoe and/or orthoses.

SHOE MODIFICATION FOR PLANTAR ULCERS

Objectives

Footwear management pedorthic care for the prevention of plantar ulcers is, in general, the same for all areas of the foot. Prescription footwear should never be considered a primary treatment for ulcers; rather, such care for ulcers is intended strictly as a long-term management technique for maintaining healed areas and preventing further ulceration. Appropriate prescription footwear is considered an important factor in this effort, particularly in the insensate foot.

The specific objectives in the pedorthic management of plantar ulcers are even distribution of plantar pressure by transfer from areas of high pressure, such as the metatarsal heads, to areas of lower pressure; shock absorption; reduction of friction and shear; by limitation of tissue motion; and accommodation of deformities.[33]

FIGURE 11
Extra-depth shoe. Cutaway shoe demonstrates shock absorption, extra-cushioned heel, and extended insole in extra-depth shoe application.

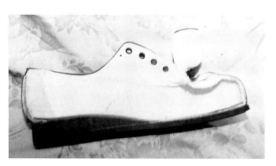

FIGURE 12
Extra-depth shoe with blucher closure.

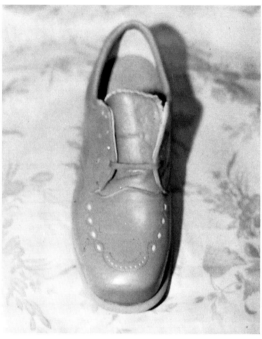

Shoes

Proper shoe fit is important in maintaining healed plantar areas and preventing further ulceration. It is crucial that the shape of the shoe match the shape of the foot. This limits overall pressure on the foot, eliminates any particular high pressure areas, and accommodates any deformities. A shoe with an extra-depth toebox (Fig. 11) or heat moldable upper may be required for more severe deformities or in cases of mismated feet. Other important characteristics for a shoe used in the pedorthic management of plantar ulcers include (1) a long medial counter to control the heel and medial arch and to decrease shear forces; (2) a blucher opening to allow easy entry into the shoe (Fig. 12); (3) a shock-absorbing sole to reduce impact shock; and (4) a low heel to decrease pressure on the metatarsal heads and the toe.

External Shoe Modifications

Addition of an appropriate rocker sole will help to reduce overall pressure and impact shock. The rocker sole can help limit motion of the joints and improve weightbearing transfer. Adding of an extended steel shank can be used to enhance the effects of the rocker sole. A negative heel rocker sole may be used to further reduce pressure and impact shock on the forefoot. However, attention also must be given to the material of the sole. Such modifications should not adversely affect shock absorption.

Orthoses

The use of a total contact insert (TCI) (Fig. 13) can be quite effective in the distribution and transfer of plantar pressure and in reduction or elimination of weightbearing from problem areas. A TCI is also useful in stabilizing or restricting joint motion. In order to provide the maximum moldability essential for achieving total contact, along with the necessary shock absorption and control, a TCI mode of multiple layers of selected density materials are most often prescribed.[34]

IN-DEPTH SHOES AND SHOE MODIFICATIONS

In-Depth Shoes

The majority of diabetic footwear prescriptions begin with an in-depth shoe. It is generally a blucher-style oxford (Fig. 12) or athletic shoe with an additional ¼- to ⅜-inch of depth throughout the shoe. This depth provides the extra volume needed to accommodate both the foot and the TCI, an orthosis that is custom-made to fit the exact contours of the individual foot. The additional depth is necessary in accommodating deformities associated with the diabetic foot, such as hammertoes and claw toes,

FIGURE 13
Total contact orthoses. **Left,** Toe filler.
Right, Total contact insole triple density
third metatarsal head ulcer.

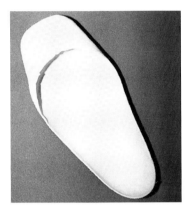

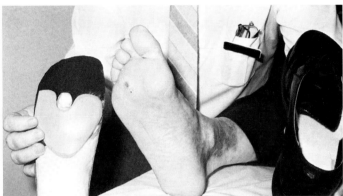

as well as moderate medial and lateral bony prominences resulting from Charcot deformities.

Other features common to the in-depth shoes that are especially useful in the care of the diabetic foot include their having lightweight, shock-absorbing soles and strong counters. In-depth shoes are made with a variety of upper materials, including deerskin and cowhide; some have a heat-moldable lining material, which allows the upper to be customized to the individual foot, a necessary consideration for severe deformities. In-depth shoes also come in a wide range of shapes and sizes to accommodate almost all feet except those with severe skeletal distortion.

External Shoe Modifications

The outside of the shoe can be modified in a variety of ways. External shoe modifications commonly prescribed for the diabetic foot include rocker soles, stabilization, extended steel shank, cushion heel, wedge, and customized upper.

Rocker Sole As its name suggests, the basic function of a rocker sole is to literally "rock" the foot from heel-strike to toe-off without bending the shoe and foot (Fig. 14). The actual shape of a rocker sole, however, varies according to the patient's specific foot problems and the desired effect of the rocker sole. In general, the biomechanical effects of a rocker sole are that it substi-tutes for lost motion in the foot and/or ankle and associated pain, deformity, or stiffness. The modification results in an overall improvement in gait and relief of pressure areas of the plantar surface.

Stabilization This involves adding material to the medial or lateral portion of the shoe in order to stabilize some part of the foot. There are two methods of stabilization: the flare and the stabilizer. A flare is an extension to the heel and/or sole of the shoe. Flares can be placed medial or lateral to stabilize a hindfoot, midfoot, or forefoot instability. A stabilizer is an additional extension added to the side of the shoe, including both the sole and upper. Made from rigid foam or crepe, a stabilizer provides more extensive control than a flare. The stabilizers are used for more severe medial or lateral instability of the hindfoot or midfoot usually in pronation.

Extended Steel Shank An extended steel shank is a strip of spring steel that is inserted between the layers of the sole, extending from the heel to the toe of the shoe (Fig. 15). Most commonly used in combination with a rocker sole, they will make the rocker sole more effective as well as decrease distortion of the rocker sole. An extended steel shank can also prevent the shoe from bending, limiting toe and midfoot motion and aiding in propulsion on toe-off.

FIGURE 14
Rocker soles. **Left,** Rocker sole (toe and heel). **Center,** Healing sandal. **Right,** Double rocker sole.

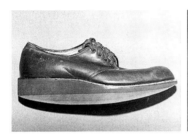
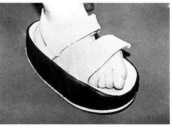
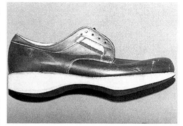

FIGURE 15
Crepe-soled shoe prepared for brace. Attachment at middle steel shank.

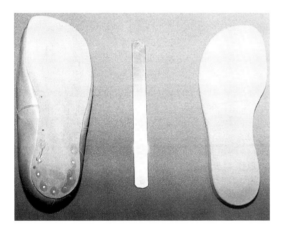

Cushion Heel A cushion heel is best achieved by a wedge of shock-absorbing material that is added between the heel and sole of the shoe. Its purpose is to provide a maximum amount of shock absorption under the heel (in addition to that provided by a total contact insert), while maintaining a stable stance.

Wedge A wedge of sole material is sometimes added medially or laterally to the heel of the shoe or occasionally to both the heel and sole (Fig. 16). It can be inserted between the upper and the sole, or it can be added directly to the bottom of the shoe to redirect the weightbearing position of the foot. A wedge can also be useful in stabilizing a flexible deformity in a corrected position or in accommodating a fixed deformity (by essentially bringing the ground to the foot).

Customized Upper Occasionally, to accommodate a severe or unusual (but often localized) foot deformity, it becomes necessary to make a shoe modification that does not fit into any of the above categories. By creating a customized shoe upper, the patient whose foot will not otherwise fit into a stock in-depth shoe can avoid the expense and delay associated with a full custom-made shoe. A Charcot foot deformity is a good example of the type that might require a customized upper or a full custom shoe.

External Shoe Modifications

Forefoot Modifications appropriate for the forefoot include the toe-only rocker sole, the negative heel rocker sole, the extended steel shank, the flare, and the customized upper.

The purpose of a toe-only rocker sole is to increase weightbearing proximal to the metatarsal heads and to reduce the need for toe dorsiflexion on toe-off. Indications for the toe-only rocker sole include metatarsal ulcers; hallux rigidus; and callus or ulcer on the distal portion of a claw, hammer, or mallet toe. Shaped with both the rocker angle at the toe and a negative heel, the combination negative heel rocker sole can relieve forefoot pressure by shifting it to the hindfoot and midfoot. It is therefore useful for prominent metatarsal heads

FIGURE 16
Wedges. **Left,** Heel wedge. **Right,** Heel wedges can be inserted between the sole or put inside the shoe.

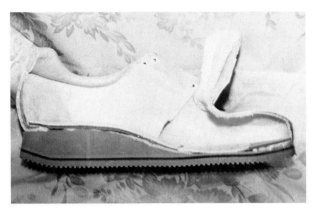

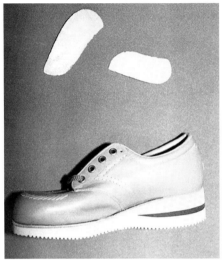

with extreme ulcers or callusing, and distal toe ulcers.

An extended steel shank is useful for hallux limitus or rigidus. The flare is used to stabilize a forefoot instability. The customized upper is useful for a severe forefoot deformity.

Midfoot Modifications appropriate for the midfoot include the double rocker sole, the heel-to-toe rocker sole, the flare-stabilizer, the medial wedge, and the custom upper. The double rocker sole has a rocker angle at both the heel and toe with the section of the sole removed in the midfoot area, thereby giving the appearance of two rocker soles—one at the hindfoot and one at the forefoot. Because the thinnest area of the double rocker sole is at the midfoot, it can be used to relieve a midfoot problem area, such as a midfoot prominence associated with a rocker bottom foot or a midfoot collapse.

When shaped with a rocker angle at both the heel and the toe, the heel-to-toe rocker sole can be used to relieve midfoot pain and to accommodate a loss of motion due to a Charcot deformity. The flare-stabilizer can control a midfoot instability. The medial wedge is used for extreme pronation and the customized upper is used for a severe deformity in the midfoot area.

Hindfoot Modifications appropriate for the hindfoot include the heel-to-toe rocker, the flare-stabilizer, and the cushion heel.

Shaped with a severe angle at both the heel and the toe, the heel-to-toe rocker sole is intended to decrease heel-strike forces on the calcaneus and decrease the need for ankle motion. It is indicated for calcaneal ulcers. The flare-stabilizer stabilizes hindfoot instability. The cushion heel is indicated for calcaneal ulcers or rigid hindfoot. The lateral wedge is used for accommodating a varus heel deformity.

CUSTOM-MADE SHOES

Custom-made shoes are indicated only for extremely severe deformities and for the foot which cannot be fit with an in-depth shoe, even with extensive modifications. In these instances, a custom-made shoe is constructed from a cast or model of the patient's foot. These rare cases include severe Charcot foot deformities and occasional partial foot amputations. Custom-made shoes should be checked periodically for fit and to determine whether the foot has undergone any significant changes.

THE OCCLUSIVE CAST

The most universally accepted treatment of diabetic foot ulcers is casting.[35-37] The principle here is the protection of the ulcer in a tissue immobilized cast, where inflammatory response and ingrowth of granulation tissue can proceed undisturbed while allowing limited safe weightbearing through more widely dispersed plantar weight distribution. Following debridement, a single sterile gauze dressing is applied to the ulcer area. If a stockinette is to be used, any folding or rolling of the gauze dressing must be carefully avoided. It is perhaps just as effective to avoid using a wound dressing. A thin layer of felt or closed cell foam may be applied to the ulcer area and windowed to avoid direct pressure on the ulcer (Fig. 17). Similarly, light felt pads are placed over bony prominences and along the tibial crest. A generous layer of cast padding is applied, again with great care to avoid the rolling or binding that could result in increased skin pressure. The use of soft roll is not universal because some centers use no cast padding at all, and the plaster is carefully applied directly to the stockinette. This is difficult, however, and requires great care and experience in cast technique.

The decision to cover the toes with the cast is based on the concept that the toes should be protected, both from direct trauma, including the cast edges, and from the possibility of foreign bodies entering the cast through the lower opening. With the open toe method, abrasion or ulceration over the dorsum of the toes at the level of the metatarsophalangeal joints will often occur. The disadvantage of covering the toes is that skin maceration may occur due to moisture accumulation. However, protection can be accomplished without covering the toes by doubling and turning the stockinette back to prevent foreign body entry. Fabrication of a sufficiently long toe opening, with the soft layer folded back, will protect the toes from direct trauma. This technique permits some circulation of air and allows the inspection of toes, if needed.

The Trilayer Covered Cast Technique

Total contact casts about the foot are best molded from rigid plaster. Generally, at least the base layer is best made of plaster. If contouring is a concern, elasticized plaster bandages can be used. When elastic type plaster is used, no tension or "stretch" should be applied when rolling the plaster, which is particularly important over the malleoli to allow immediate ambulation. The cast is then reinforced and finished with fiberglass. The surface of fiberglass is quite rough, making it mandatory to protect the opposite foot, particularly the surface of the opposing medial malleolus. This can be accomplished by wearing a knee-high athletic sock on the uncasted leg. In addition, the cast may be covered with stockinette as a precaution. If fiberglass is used, great attention must be given to the cast margins because of potential skin abrasion. The diabetic patient heals poorly, even at the upper calf, and skin ulcers are difficult to heal.

Slipper-type casts should never be used because rolling at the malleoli and shifting at the calcaneus can lead to skin breakdown. Further, in an asensory foot, there is the concern that foreign bodies may enter the cast and remain undetected.

The technique for applying a short leg trilayer occlusive cast is outlined as follows.

Layer I: A tubular stockinette is applied over a freshly debrided wound without dressing with care taken to avoid folds or twists. The toe end is left longer than full length, and then is rolled as it later will be used to cover the cast. A ⅛-inch piece of felt is cut to provide a window at the ulcerated area. A full plantar piece is applied. Contoured felt is placed about the heel and the malleoli. A narrow piece of felt is also placed along the full length of the tibial crest to protect it. Soft cast padding may be applied to position the felt and to protect the remaining soft tissues, including the toes; however, many institutions use no cast padding at all. Cotton padding is often placed between each toe.

Layer II: A plaster-of-paris cast is fashioned about the foot and the lower portion of the calf with care taken to mold the contours of the foot.

FIGURE 17
Cast application. **Top left,** Midfoot Wagner 2 ulcer complicating midfoot osteoarthropathy. **Top right,** Application of cut-out felt pad. Note the ulcer marked on stockinette. **Bottom left,** Elastic type plaster base coat application over soft-cast padding. Note excess stockinette for outside cast protection. **Bottom right,** Finished fiberglass cast with stockinette and rocker sole cast boot for ambulation. Note the twist closure of stockinette at toe.

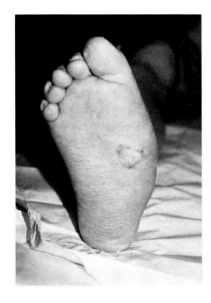
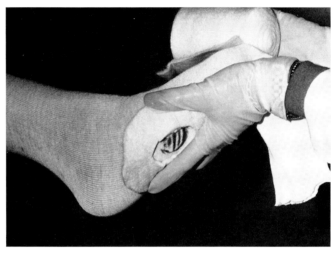
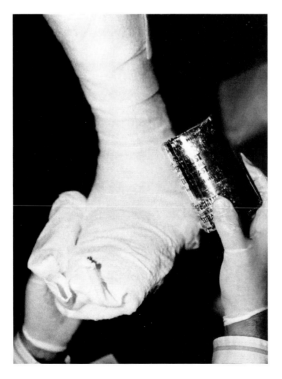
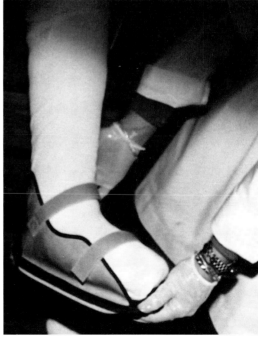

Layer III: Fiberglass is used to complete the calf portion of the cast and it is extended at least 1 inch beyond all toes. Compression of the toes or infolding of the underlying plaster should be avoided.

Covering: The covering, consisting of the extra stockinette at the toe, can then be unrolled and twisted twice to form an occlusive barrier at the toes. The remainder then is folded back to entirely cover the fiberglass cast up to its proximal portion. This, when allowed to adhere to the drying fiberglass, will form a cast covering, which helps protect the opposite foot from abrasion.

The alternative is to carefully mold the cast closed at the toes, avoiding any compression. If the occlusive regular plaster technique is used, a covering, while helpful, is unnecesssary. Although either a cast "heel" or a rocker created with fiberglass may be used, a cast shoe with shock absorption and rocker effect is preferred. Ambulation is allowed as soon as the cast dries. The cast is changed weekly initially, and then every 2 or 3 weeks until healing is evident. Cast changes may be more frequent if drainage from the ulcer is significant.

Most occlusive casts are applied in anticipation that they will not bear weight. The reality, however, is that most casts seem to be used for bearing weight, especially if the diabetic patient has visual problems, is older, or obese, or finds it difficult to use crutches. Thus, it is advisable to fashion the cast to bear weight, although this is certainly the less desirable option for a plantar ulcer.

Most clinics supply the patient with a weight-bearing-type boot over a fiberglass-reinforced plaster cast (Fig. 18). Walker cast heels probably should be avoided because they create high stresses in the area immediately above their placement and can result in angular forces if malposition exists.

Use of a Cast Brace

A removable cast brace can be used for both diabetic ulcer care and in management of osteoarthropathy (Fig. 18). When used in the diabetic neuropathic patient, such devices must be protectively padded, cautiously fitted, and closely monitored (Outlines 4 and 5). The trauma-type cast brace is not optimum for such efforts, and

---

OUTLINE 4
Objectives of cast bracing of the diabetic ulcer

1. To control heel and foot position
2. To achieve reduced pressure from breakdown area
3. With custom insole, to allow pressure transfer
4. In the Charcot foot, to facilitate immobilization

OUTLINE 5
Indications for use in diabetes

1. To control joint motion in Charcot osteoarthropathy of the hindfoot and ankle
2. In diabetic foot ulcers of the plantar aspect of the foot, as an interval measure
3. For treatment of diabetic foot ulcers when wound care is needed
4. For frequent evaluations in infected diabetic foot ulcers as an adjunctive management

---

requires custom cushioning for safe use in the insensate foot. A closed heel type cast brace may be used with a dressing like a cast.

The typical "posttrauma" cast walker can be modified with pads for the use with a supportive device for patients with diabetic osteoarthropathy of the hindfoot and ankle. The adjustable ankle type of brace is suitable for patients with altered ankle position and, with custom padding, can be safely used to control motion of the hindfoot and ankle. Such a device may be used primarily in lieu of casting or as an interim device between casting and shoe brace. The posttraumatic cast brace is suitable only for those patients with relatively anatomic talotibial positioning.

Recently, a new design in cast bracing has become available with a closed padded heel. This fixed ankle heel control type cast brace may be modified for use in diabetic foot ulcers and midfoot collapse secondary to Charcot osteoarthropathy. These cast braces offer the advantage over plaster type casts in that they may be

FIGURE 18
Left, Post trauma-type cast brace. Use of multiple inserts with standard cast brace with adjustable ankle type used in ankle stabilization. **Right,** Fixed ankle-type cast brace with heel control used with custom orthotic for both ulcer management and osteoarthropathy.

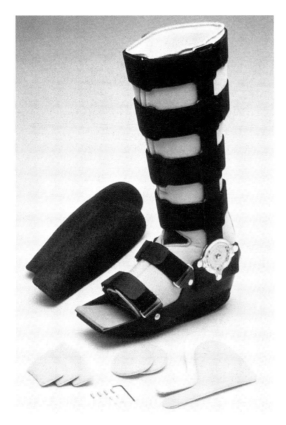
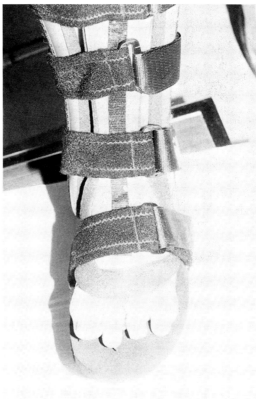

removed for wound care, such as soaks, and permit for easy, frequent inspection of suspected infections. Further advantages are, of course, better hygiene and patient comfort. This cast brace is designed to control heel position and foot motion. Thus, only the contoured closed back design provides for acceptable heel control to avoid shear in the diabetic patient. This type of walker, if carefully fitted, will maintain the position of the total contact insole.

The fixed ankle/heel control types are finding application as an interval step between total contact casts and custom shoe wear. However, custom fitting of insoles is a necessity if satisfac-tory ulcer prevention and ulcer treatment are to be achieved.

Posttrauma cast brace can be fit with pads, arch supports, and modified to accept dressings. The fixed ankle/heel control type can be used with custom insole.

FOLLOW-UP

The frequency of cast changes usually de-pends on the size of the ulcer and the amount of drainage and swelling of the extremity. Swelling will dissipate rapidly after the first application of a cast, which then may need to be changed as soon as 3 days. Subsequently, casts can be changed less frequently. A patient's understanding of the problem and compliance with instructions as well as the progress of the ulcer determine the follow-up schedule. Most authors suggest that the cast be changed monthly; as frequently as every 3 weeks for the more acute inflammatory type problem or as infrequently as every 6 weeks for a long-term granulating ulcer.

At each cast change, the ulcer is again debrided, measured, and documented. If healing does not progress, the physician should re-evaluate the vascular status and consider other alternatives, such as hyperbaric oxygen (see *Hyperbaric Oxygen*). Faced with treatment failure and progression of the ulcer, amputation not only will avoid the potential of further complications, such as deep-seated infection or distant abscess, but may improve the patient's life-style and may be more psychologically acceptable to both the patient and the care providers (see *Amputation Surgery*).

 ## HEEL ULCERS

Perhaps the most difficult ulcers to manage are those of the heel. The anatomic contour promotes distraction of tissues after breakdown begins. The subcutaneous fat pad over the calcaneus offers little support for a granulation tissue base and, once exposed, is the source of constant drainage and effusion. The anatomic dependent position of the heel in bed is a pressure threat to even any conservative effort. The pooling effect of lymphatic and venous supply enhances tissue edema. The heel has an end arterial-type blood supply, which, even in healthy individuals, contributes to delayed wound healing.

Once established, the heel ulcer usually requires extensive anatomic resection and a regional reconstruction. Osteomyelitis is relatively common and once established, the bony architecture of the calcaneus offers little architectural defense to its spread. Successful treatment necessitates removal of not only all infected bone, but of sufficient bone to allow easy skin closure without tension at the skin margins.[38]

WOUND RISK FACTORS

A protocol of follow-up for the foot at risk has been developed and is used in foot-at-risk clinics, such as St. Michael's Hospital, Milwaukee, Wisconsin. Each patient is assigned a risk category, which determines the return appointment and general education required.

An understanding of risk factors helps when determining the appropriate approach to wound management and control of infection. A diabetic foot ulcer with chronic open drainage and persistent serum contamination is an ideal site for the introduction of superficial and deep infections. Further complicating such risks are the underlying factors that render the diabetic wound more prone to infection; vascularly, the presence of large-vessel atherosclerosis secondary to the diabetic process, in combination with small-vessel disease, compromises circulation. The endocrine imbalance further compromises response by the reticuloendothelial system compromising wound healing even at the cellular level. The clinical approach must be tailored to all of the individual problems.

In general, the long-term nutritional endocrine imbalance leads to an increased incidence of large-vessel disease and small-vessel disease. As noted above, this is the result of basement membrane change in arterioles, adversely affecting circulation. Increased cellular oxygenation demand secondary to changes in metabolism then furthers the oxygen deprivation. Decreased oxygen adversely affects leukocyte mobility, and the hyperglycemia favors bacterial growth. The net result is that the compromised tissue response favors necrotic deterioration, resulting in ulceration and tissue death.

Hydrostatic pressure, however, is perhaps the most significant factor in persistent effusion and tissue edema. The dependent position of the lower limbs promotes tissue congestion and compromises healing. Although diabetic wound problems do occur in the younger patient, such wounds are usually dry. It is more common for both the superficial necrotic-type ulcer and deep-seated infection to be found in the older diabetic patient with deteriorated venous and lymphatic systems, which increase interstitial fluid pressure and create static edema. In addition to these superficial tissue problems, a compartment syndrome may occur within the midfoot. Inflammation and edema can increase intracompartment pressure, causing vascular blockage, which further compromises circulation and leads to intrinsic muscle necrosis and fibrosis in the midfoot compartment that further impair distal circulation.

In evaluation of the diabetic ulcer, the physician should be concerned as to whether infection is present.[39] The differentiation between surface contamination of a diabetic foot ulcer and true infection is frequently unclear. The diagnosis of infection cannot be based strictly on culture, but rather must take into account both clinical evaluation, as well as the type and amount of drainage, and the surrounding inflammation, and temperature, in addition to laboratory screening. Most ulcers contain a mixed flora of bacteria, and rarely is a culture of the uncomplicated ulcer necessary.

When infection is present, the multiplicity of organisms in diabetic wounds, particularly coliform organisms, can lead to gas formation in soft tissue, which on radiographs may suggest *Clostridium*-type gas gangrene. *Clostridium* infections, however, are uncommon in the diabetic foot; even if there is radiographic evidence of large formations of gas in soft tissue, it usually stems from mixed coliform infections. Infection is often suspected, but rarely found, in diabetic neuroarthropathy. Swelling and warmth associated with radiographic findings of marked bone absorption and bone destruction in the foot can present a diagnostic dilemma, particularly when diabetes is mild or undiagnosed.

 INFECTIONS

Foot infections in diabetic patients present a special challenge to treatment. Foot infection is the most common admitting diagnosis for diabetic patients in the hospital.[40] Because these infections may cause few symptoms, patients with foot infections often delay seeking medical care. In one study of patients with serious foot infections, the average time before referral was 23 weeks, with 60% of patients receiving only oral antibiotics during that time.[41] Additional

diabetic complications, such as immune system deficiencies, neuropathy, and vascular insufficiency often combine to allow rapid progression in many cases. The ability to make an appropriate diagnosis is complicated by misleading culture results and radiographic findings that are often nonspecific. Overdiagnosis can also occur as it is sometimes difficult to differentiate acute neuroarthropathic changes from infection. A thorough understanding of the nature of diabetic foot infections is necessary to be able to rapidly institute a rational treatment plan in these patients.

There are conflicting opinions in the medical literature as to whether diabetic patients have an increased susceptibility to infection. The authors of some studies have reported that there is no convincing evidence that immunologic competence is impaired in diabetics.[42-47] Other reports indicate an increased frequency of infection and impaired leukocyte function and mobility in these patients.[48-54] Clinical experience suggests that diabetic patients are at increased risk for developing a foot infection compared to nondiabetic patients. Predisposing factors resulting in noncompliance with treatment include poor visual acuity, making routine foot inspection unreliable; peripheral neuropathy, which leads to insensibility with delays in diagnosis and treatment; and cutaneous lesions, which act as portals of entry for bacteria. Skin lesions that belong in this category include fissures in dry skin and the margin of callouses as well as ulcers that result from ill-fitting shoes. These problems are much more frequent in poorly controlled patients than in well-controlled individuals.

Microbiologic studies have shown that different areas of the leg and foot can be colonized by different types of microorganisms. In barefoot individuals, the lower leg has a relatively low bacterial count due to the relatively cool and dry conditions in this area, the impermeability of the thickened stratum corneum, and the presence of antimicrobial metabolic products of the skin.[55] Because shoes retain moisture against the skin, there is increased bacterial colonization; the density of bacteria in the toe webs can exceed 1 million/cm². Despite the fact that the feet of diabetic patients are generally drier than in persons without diabetes (because of impaired

FIGURE 19
Left, Lateral radiograph of the foot showing a foreign body in the sole.

Right, MRI of the same foot showing the area of abscess.

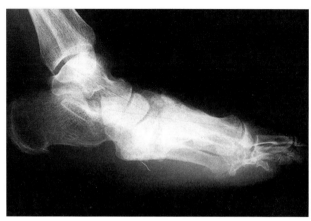
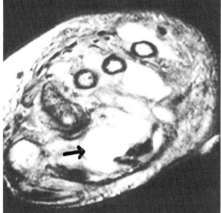

sweating associated with peripheral neuropathy), diabetic feet are colonized by the same flora as in persons without diabetes.[56]

Several types of significant infections occur in the feet of diabetics, including cellulitis, abscess of the deep compartments of the foot, and infections associated with neuropathic ulcers. Foot infections are almost always caused by local invasion rather than hematogenous spread. An infection that begins with a minor penetrating trauma, such as stepping on a thin wooden splinter or metal pin, can rapidly progress to a deep abscess (Fig. 19). This kind of infection is particularly common in patients who have peripheral neuropathy and diminished plantar sensation. Visual inspection of the foot may reveal nothing more than a pinpoint mark on the sole as evidence that there has been perforating trauma. Foreign bodies retained in the soft tissues of the foot should be considered indicative of this type of trauma. Patients may complain of nothing more than the acute onset of swelling in the foot. Although they may have neuropathy and diminished cutaneous sensation, perception of deep pain is frequently preserved, and patients may note discomfort in the foot, especially with weightbearing. Physical examination is remarkable for dorsal midfoot swelling, occasionally with plantar fullness that obscures the lon-

gitudinal arch. Associated cellulitis may be confined to the foot or it may ascend the leg. Common systemic manifestations of infection include fever, elevated white blood cell count with a left shift, and increased insulin requirements. Blood cultures should be obtained in these patients, especially during fever "spikes," where there is a transient bacteremia.

Any patient suspected of having a deep abscess should be examined immediately by an orthopaedic surgeon. If the clinician is confident in the diagnosis (eg, presence of pus and a cavity that can be probed with a cotton-tipped applicator), the patient should be brought to the operating room for drainage of the abscess following a rapid but thorough workup. Tests should include a complete blood count with differential, erythrocyte sedimentation rate, chemistries, and urinalysis. In one study, however, leukocytosis was absent in 26% of diabetic patients with infection.[57] Preoperative plain radiographic evaluation should include three views of the foot (anteroposterior, oblique, and lateral) with a careful search for foreign bodies and evidence of osteomyelitis.

Computed tomography (CT) scan with soft-tissue windows is helpful in assessing the location and extent of the abscess cavity. Magnetic resonance imaging (MRI) is the imaging modality of choice in the preoperative assessment of deep abscesses of the foot. It allows excellent resolution of the details of soft-tissue anatomy and provides an assessment of contiguous bony structures for osteomyelitis. A foot abscess is a surgical emergency and drainages should not be unduly delayed in order to obtain these tests.

Thirteen percent of patients hospitalized for diabetic foot problems have osteomyelitis.[58] Often, it is a chronic plantar ulcer that acts as the portal of entry for bacterial osteomyelitis. A study of 41 foot ulcers reported that 68% had osteomyelitis by indepth evaluation with indium 111.[59] With time, these ulcers become colonized with mixed bacterial flora, which spread to the periosteum and joints along fascial and soft-tissue planes. The greater the size and depth of the ulcer, the more likely the risk of underlying osteomyelitis. It has been suggested that an ulcer with bone exposed by inspection or probe has a 100% incidence of osteomyelitis, and that an ulcer more than 2 cm in diameter has a 94% incidence of bone infection.[60] It is unclear how long an ulcer must be present to subject the patient to a significant risk of osteomyelitis. Clearly, the sooner an ulcer is healed, the less likely it is to cause bone infection.

There are several ways to determine if a neuropathic ulcer is infected or is complicated by an underlying abscess or osteomyelitis. If a patient with a long-standing, previously indolent appearing ulcer presents with the acute onset of swelling and erythema in the foot and with purulent, foul-smelling drainage from that ulcer, a deep infection is present. Plain radiographs should be obtained to look for signs of soft-tissue abscess, osteomyelitis, or a foreign body. Frank pus must be considered a surgical emergency and preoperative evaluation may include an MRI of the foot. This allows good delineation of the extent of the cavity as well as the pattern of loculation that may be present. Additionally, the MRI aids in determining which bones and joints are involved in the infectious process and which structures are necrotic. Surgical planning should allow placement of incisions dorsally, medially, or laterally if possible to avoid plantar incisions. All purulent material must be excised, along with any foreign body that may be present. Initial debridement should be performed without a tourniquet inflated and should include the excision of all infected and necrotic tissue. Tissue that is questionably viable should be preserved for a "second look" operation at 48 hours. After adequate debridement, closure over drains then can be performed by direct skin closure or a free-tissue transfer can be performed.

Determining whether a chronic plantar ulcer is infected is a difficult task. Deciding if it is associated with an underlying osteomyelitis is even more challenging. Every ulcer will drain small amounts of serous fluid on the dressing that covers it because of the loss of overlying integument. Generally this is straw-colored material, which is not malodorous. Excessive drainage, especially if it is malodorous, is usually a sign that the ulcer is infected. If the remainder of the foot examination does not reveal unusual swelling or ascending cellulitis, out-patient treatment is instituted, provided the patient is reliable and can be monitored regularly.

Superficial cultures of the surface of the ulcer can be misleading in predicting the infecting organism. The most reliable method by which to determine the etiology of the infection is to obtain deep cultures in the operating room through an incision placed through uninvolved skin. This subjects the patient to a surgical procedure, however, and may not be cost-effective. Deep aerobic, anaerobic, and fungal cultures are adequate in most cases for determining the causative microorganisms. The ulcer should first be cleansed mechanically with a hexidine solution and then irrigated with sterile saline. The skin around the ulcer should be painted with a povidone-iodine solution and then the deep culture obtained. In one series, 50% of wounds contained three or more microorganisms and more than 60% of wounds had two or more.[57] A recent study suggests that 74% of intraoperative cultures contain diphtheroids.[61] Because such a high percentage of foot infections involve mixed bacterial flora, anaerobic cultures also must be obtained. Anaerobic infection must be considered present in any patient with foul-smelling drainage. Knowledge and experience dealing with diabetic infections are necessary in interpreting the culture results. For example, typical skin flora can cause deep infections, and deciding if an organism is a contaminant is sometimes difficult. Conversely, certain bacteria rarely associated with significant infections, such as coagulase-negative Staphylococcus and Streptococcus viridans, may be the responsible microorganism in serious diabetic infections. When cultured, these microorganisms cannot be dismissed as contaminants. Treating every isolated microorganism with an antibiotic is difficult and usually unnecessary, however. If there is a question in interpreting the results of the culture, consultation with an infectious disease specialist is recommended.

INFECTION DIAGNOSIS

Several important radiologic aids can assist the clinician in making the diagnosis of osteomyelitis. Conventional radiographs take at least 2 weeks to show the bony changes associated with acute osteomyelitis, most commonly, periosteal reaction, cortical erosions, or lytic lesions. Occasionally, a pathologic fracture may be found at the site of osteomyelitis. Chronic osteomyelitis may not be revealed on plain film examination. CT has limited value in diagnosing osteomyelitis, but can be used preoperatively to evaluate the extent of soft-tissue and bony involvement. High-resolution CT scanning can identify subtle cortical irregularities before they can be seen on plain radiographs. Neither conventional radiographs nor CT scans are helpful in differentiating osteomyelitis from Charcot neuroarthropathy. Both pathologic conditions may demonstrate radiographic evidence of osteopenia, bone destruction, and fragmentation. Scintigraphy can be used for differentiation. Technetium-99m methylenediphosphonate scanning is a very sensitive tool in detecting osteomyelitis; however, it is a relatively nonspecific test because cellulitis, osteomyelitis, fracture, and Charcot neuroarthropathy will result in uptake on the bone scan. In addition, the scans can be negative in culture-positive infection in the presence of concurrent vascular insufficiency. Reliance solely on the bone scan to determine the presence of osteomyelitis will result in an excessively high false-positive rate and treatment of many diabetic feet for infection that have other noninfectious inflammatory processes; ie, Charcot fracture.

Combining technetium scanning with indium-111-labeled leukocyte scanning is the most accurate method of determining the presence of osseous involvement. The indium scan is performed by withdrawing 50 ml of blood from the patient, treating it to tag the leukocyte with radioactive indium isotope, and then reinfusing the blood. The leukocytes accumulate at the site of infection carrying the radionuclide with them and the patient is then scanned. It is very sensitive and specific for acute osteomyelitis, but may be less so with chronic cases, especially when the infectious agent elicits little response from acute inflammatory cells (leukocytes); for example, in chronic nonsuppurative tuberculous osteomyelitis, in which the predominant cell is the monocyte.

A relative disadvantage to indium scanning is that the radioactive emission is low, resulting in poorer resolution as compared to technetium scanning. For this reason, the bone scan is usually combined with the indium scan. The clinician can localize the increased uptake on the bone scan and decide whether it represents infection or some other inflammatory process by comparing it to the indium scan.

Caution must be exercised in the interpretation of the indium scan. Because acute inflammation will cause a hyperemic response with a relative increased concentration of leukocytes, the indium scan may appear weakly positive in cases of intense, noninfectious inflammatory conditions. Relying solely on these tests may result in inappropriate treatment, thus evaluation of results must be tempered by clinical judgment. Under current investigation is a preparation of a technetium-labeled antibody that has specific binding affinity for an antigen on the leukocyte. A patient with suspected osteomyelitis would receive an intravenous administration of this material and be scanned 1 hour later. The advantages are the attainment of rapid results, a high sensitivity and specificity for infection, and a much higher resolution than indium scans. It is currently undergoing clinical trials.

MRI resonance imaging is also useful for assessing osteomyelitis. In one study, MRI had a 99% sensitivity, 81% specificity, and 94% accuracy in detecting osteomyelitis.[62] Superior soft-tissue definition and sensitivity make MRI an excellent tool for preoperatively assessing the diabetic foot. Disadvantages, in addition to its cost, include its relatively low specificity and the difficulty in determining the true extent of osseous involvement, because, in many cases, surrounding noninfected marrow edema cannot be differentiated from osteomyelitis. MRI using gadolinium contrast may have an important role in selecting which patients will benefit from intravenous antibiotic therapy alone or which patients will require surgical ablation followed by antimicrobial coverage as the best solution for treating their bone infection. Because gadolinium is given intravenously it accumulates in areas of edema. If an area of osteomyelitis does not enhance with gadolinium, there may not be adequate circulation to support appropriate tissue levels of antibiotic, and surgical resection would be the treatment of choice. If the bone enhances with contrast, however, it may be possible to attain sufficiently high antibiotic titers to treat the osteomyelitis medically with a good chance of success.

INFECTION TREATMENT

If the diabetic patient is reliable, afebrile, otherwise healthy and has well-controlled blood sugar levels, a decision may be made regarding appropriate outpatient antibiotic management. The foot must not have deep soft-tissue infection, osteomyelitis, or gangrene. Ascending cellulitis and significant swelling are also relative contraindications to outpatient therapy. Broad-spectrum antimicrobial agents should be instituted initially pending culture results. Combination drug therapy may provide better coverage than single oral agents. The antibiotic chosen should be bactericidal rather than bacteriostatic because of possible defects in leukocyte function. Large doses of antibiotic often must be used to achieve high tissue concentrations because tissue perfusion is often poor. The length of antibiotic treatment is tailored to the individual situation; however, a good rule of thumb is to continue treatment for 14 days for soft-tissue infections and 6 weeks if there is bone involvement. Following the complete resection of all infected bone, antibiotics may be continued for a period of 2 weeks.

Several drugs are commonly used in the outpatient management of infections of the diabetic foot. Although not intended to be all-inclusive, common antibiotics are listed in Table 4.

Several outpatient drug regimens can be used to treat diabetic foot infections. Oral clindamycin or cephalexin for 2 weeks has been shown to be effective treatment in a selected group of patients.[63] Combination therapy is more commonly employed; examples include clindamycin plus ciprofloxacin, ciprofloxacin plus metronidazole, or ampicillin-clavulanate plus clindamycin or metronidazole. Clindamycin (Cleocin) plus ciprofloxacin (Cipro) is particularly effective in providing broad-spectrum coverage against gram-positive, gram-negative, and anaerobic organisms. Therapy should be continued for at least 2 weeks with significant improvement noted by 5 days. Patients who do not respond appropriately should be hospitalized for further evaluation and the administration of parenteral antibiotics. There should be no hesitancy in trying to decide whether a patient is responding favorably to outpatient treatment. Any patient who has failed to progress should be hospitalized.

The success of outpatient therapy depends on patient compliance, appropriate assistance at home, limb elevation, and proper local wound care. It is better not to use occlusive type dressings in the presence of infection and drainage. Frequent absorbent dressing changes should be performed. Judicious ulcer debridement should be performed by the physician, as needed. Careful monitoring and assessment are necessary because these infections can progress rapidly despite oral therapy.

ADJUNCTIVE TREATMENT

Hospitalization and intravenous antibiotics are required for any patient who is noncompliant, acutely ill or toxic, or has an infection complicated by excessive swelling, ascending cellulitis, deep soft-tissue involvement, osteomyelitis, or gangrene. Hospitalization may be indicated in patients with known borderline circulation to their feet presenting with acute infection. In the noninfectious resting state, the circulation may be merely adequate to support the tissues of the foot. With infection, the increased metabolic demands of the tissues render the existing blood flow inadequate with the potential development of gangrene. Careful monitoring is imperative. The use of adjunctive hyperbaric oxygen (the intermittent administration of 100% oxygen inhaled at a pressure greater than sea level) should

TABLE 4
Drugs used in the outpatient management of the diabetic foot

Antibiotic	Dosage	Target	Side Effects
Clindamycin (Cleocin)	300 mg po qid	Most gram-postitive cocci and anaerobic organisms (specifically, *Staphylococcus aureus*, *S epidermidis*, streptococci, and pneumococci) Most gram-positive and gram-negative anaerobic organisms (including *Bacteriodes*, *Fusobacterium*, *Propionibacterium*, *Peptococcus*, and *Peptostreptococcus* sp) *Clostridium* usually sensitive, but susceptibility testing is recommended Not effective against gram-negative rod bacteria	Severe colitis
Ampicillin-clavulanate (Augmentin)	500 mg po tid	*Staphylococcus aureus* (beta-lactamase—producing and non-beta-lacatamase—producing), *S epidermidis*, *Enterococcus*, and *Pneumococcus* A wide range of gram-negative rods as well as the anaerobe The treatment of skin infections caused by *S aureus*, *Escherichia coli*, and *Klebsiella*	Hypersensitivity reactions, pseudomembranous colitis Diarrhea in 9% of individuals
Ciprofloxacin (Cipro)	750 mg po bid	*Staphylococcus aureus* and gram-negative rods, including *Pseudomonas aeruginosa* specifically, (against methicillin-susceptible and methicillin-resistant *S aureus*, *S epidermidis*, and *Pneumococcus*). Most strains of *Streptococcus aureus* are only moderately susceptible Many infections caused by gram-negative organisms, including *Pseudomonas aeruginosa*. Other *Pseudomonas* and anaerobic organisms are resistant to this agent	

TABLE 4 (continued)

Antibiotic	Dosage	Target	Side Effects
Metronidazole (Flagyl)	500 mg po tid	Anaerobic species including *Bacteroides, Fusobacterium, Clostridium, Peptococcus,* and *Peptostreptococcus*	A peripheral neuropathy, which may not be recognized in a diabetic patient with an existing neuropathy; a worsening neuropathy in a patient on this agent requires prompt discontinuation of therapy
Cephalexin (Keflex)	500 mg po qid	Staphylococci, streptococci, *Escherichia coli, Proteus mirabilis, Haemophilus influenzae,* and *Proteus mirabilis* Not active against enterococci, *Morganella morganii, Proteus vulgaris,* or *Pseudomonas*	Reactions of cephalexin with Clinitest tablets have been observed giving a false-positive test for glucose in the urine

be considered during the acute phase of infection. Limb-sized oxygen chambers or topical oxygen therapy have no role in the treatment of the diabetic foot. The increased arterial oxygen found in hyperbaric oxygen therapy serves two important roles: to support the tissues during time of relatively diminished blood flow and to boost the ability of the immune system to combat the infection. Leukocytes kill most effectively when supplied with increased amounts of oxygen.[64,65]

Antibiotic-impregnated polymethylmethacrylate spacers may also be useful adjuncts to treat infection in diabetic feet after local resection of bone. They are particularly helpful after resection of joints (ie, first metatarsophalangeal joint) when distal salvage is possible. The spacer not only delivers a high concentration of antibiotic, but also maintains appropriate tissue tension to prevent deformity of the bone deficient region. After joint resection and debridement, the spacer is prepared by mixing 1.2 g of tobramycin with one packet of polymethylmethacrylate cement.

INTRAVENOUS TREATMENT

Several intravenously administered antibiotics are effective in treating diabetic foot infections. Knowledge of their antimicrobial coverage and major route of excretion is important in selection and usage. In addition, it must be kept in mind that the concentrations of the antibiotic in bone represent only a fraction of its level in serum; for example, the concentration of cefoxitin in bone is 15% to 21%; gentamycin, 30%; and clindamycin, 29% to 49%.

Detailed descriptions of individual intravenously administered antibiotics is beyond the scope of this monograph, however, several therapeutic regimens are commonly employed in the treatment of diabetic foot infections. These are listed below.

1. Vancomycin, 1g q 12 h. Gentamycin dosage is based on body weight and renal function, Metronidazole (Flagyl) 500 mg q 8 h. Vancomycin is the antimicrobial of choice for methicillin-resistant *Staphylococcus* infection.

2. Ticarcillin-clavulanate (Timentin), 3.1 g q 4 h. Antimicrobial activity covers *S aureus, S epidermidis, Streptococcus* sp, gram-negative bacteria, including *Pseudomonas aeruginosa, Bacteroides* sp, *Clostridium* sp, and *Peptostreptococcus* sp. Because Ticarcillin is a penicillin derivative, it is contraindicated in patients who have a hypersensitivity reaction to any of the penicillins. Relative disadvantages include its frequent administration and cost.

3. Ampicillin-sulbactam (Unasyn), 3 g q 6 h. Antimicrobial activity covers *Staphylococcus aureus, S epidermidis, Streptococcus* sp, *Escherichia coli, Hemophilus influenzae, Klebsiella* sp *Proteus mirabilis, P vulgaris, Morganella morganii, Neisseria gonorrhoeae, Bacteroides* sp, *Clostridium* sp, and *Peptostreptococcus* sp. It does not have antibacterial action against *Pseudomonas* sp.

4. Impenem-cilastatin (Primaxin) 0.5 g q 6 h. Coverage is similar to that of Ticarcillin-clavulanate.

5. Cefazolin (Ancef) plus metronidazole (Flagyl).

6. Ciprofloxacin (Cipro) plus clindamycin (Cleocin).

The selection of antibiotics is often based on regional experience with respect to sensitivity and, as with most pharmaceutical regimens, is subject to rapid change. Recent monographs on orthopaedic infections would suggest certain general protocols (Table 5).

Infection that occurs in the dysvascular foot is particularly difficult to treat. Without appropriate treatment these infections are life-threatening as well as limb-threatening. A major risk factor for amputation in the face of foot infection is absence of a dorsalis pedis pulse.[66] Patients who show signs of toxicity with an infected foot and poor peripheral circulation may be candidates for immediate major amputation. Arterial Doppler evaluation should be performed to determine whether a pulse is present because swelling can easily mask the pulse by palpation. If

limb salvage is to be attempted, patients should be treated initially by bed rest, local debridement, wound care, and broad-spectrum antibiotics. Once the infection is controlled, revascularization of the limb should be considered. In one study, 98% limb salvage was demonstrated at 36 months using this protocol.[67] The morbidity of this disease is significant. In this same study, the average length of stay of the initial hospitalization was 30 days, and 31 subsequent foot procedures and 35 rehospitalizations were required in the group of 52 patients treated this way. Incidence of graft failure was 3.6% and the mortality rate was 1.8%. The authors concluded that bypass grafting is efficacious and safe as long as infection is adequately controlled first.

Diabetic foot infections are serious, often rapidly progressive conditions that require a high index of suspicion and careful patient monitoring. Patient selection is crucial in determining which infections can be managed in an outpatient setting. Appropriate antibiotic selection covering aerobic and anaerobic organisms is important in managing the infection. Radiologic assessment utilizing technetium bone and indium scanning helps confirm the diagnosis of osteomyelitis, especially when it occurs concurrently with neuroarthropathic changes. Adjuncts to treatment, such as hyperbaric oxygen and revascularization, can bring about limb salvage in selected patients.

AMPUTATION SURGERY

PREOPERATIVE EVALUATION

The foot should be examined systematically and the plantar weightbearing surfaces analyzed. The extent of infection and the neurovascular status must be assessed. The essential points on examination—other than obvious infection, ulcers, fissures, and gangrene—are the color, temperature, and nutritional state of the skin.

A level of amputation should be selected that is likely to result in recovery with a functional plantigrade foot. In amputations that result from trauma, tumor, or congenital anomalies, length is preserved at the most appropriate level consistent with prosthetic rehabilitation. In amputa-

TABLE 5
Antimicrobial therapy for osteomyelitis

Pathogen	Preferred Therapy	Dosage	Comments
Gram-positive *S aureus* (methicillin susceptible)	**β-lactamase-resistant penicillin** Nafcillin	 2 g intravenously every 6 hours	Vancomycin for penicillin
	Oxacillin	2 g intravenously every 6 hours	
	First-generation cephalosporin Cefazolin	 2 g intravenously every 8 hours	Rare cross-reaction in penicillin hypersensitivity
	Second-generation cephalosporin **Oral fluoroquinolones**	1.5 g intravenously every 8 hours	Rare cross-reaction in penicillin hypersensitivity Questionable efficacy for *S aureus*, emergence of resistance
	Ciprofloxacin	750 mg orally every 12 hours	
	Ofloxacin	400 mg orally every 12 hours	
S aureus (methicillin resistant) *S epidermidis* (methicillin resistant)	Vancomycin	1 g intravenously every 12 hours	Possible rifampin combination
Gram-negative *P aeruginosa*	**Third-generation cephalosporin** Ceftazidime	 2 g intravenously every 12 hours	 Same strains resistant
	Cefoperazone	2 g intravenously every 12 hours	
	Carbepenem Imipenem-cilastatin	 0.5 g intravenously every 6 hours	 CNS toxicity with decreased renal function
	Monobactam Aztreonam	 2 g intravenously every 8 hours	 No cross reaction in penicillin hypersensitive
	Oral fluoroquinolones		Broad spectrum, effective in long-term treatment regimens
	Ciprofloxacin	750 mg orally every 12 hours	
	Semisynthetic penicillin Piperacillin	 3 g intravenously every 6 hours	If resistant or penicillin hypersensitive, use third-generation cephalosporins, carbepenem, or monobactam

TABLE 5 (*continued*)

Pathogen	Preferred Therapy	Dosage	Comments
	Mezlocillin	3 g intravenously every 6 hours	
	Aminoglycoside		
	Amikacin	16 mg/kg/day	For highly resistant strains
	Tobramycin	5 mg/kg/day	
Entero-bacteriaceae and other gram-negatives	**Third-generation cephalosporin or oral fluoroquinolone or β-lactamase inhibitor**		
	Ticarcillin and clavulanate	3.1 g intravenously every 6 hours	Proved in mixed infection
	Carbepenem		
	Imipenem-cilastatin	0.5 g intravenously every 6 hours	Proved in mixed infection
Anaerobes	**Clindamycin**	0.9 g intravenously every 8 hours	Anti-staphylococcal activity
	Metronidazole	0.5 g intravenously every 8 hours	Anaerobic activity only

tions that result from diabetes or dysvascular foot problems, however, no well-defined criteria exist. The level of amputation is determined by functional considerations, the presence of infection, the status of the circulation, and the age and activity level of the patient.[68,69]

PREOPERATIVE CONTROL

Surgery in the face of sepsis is always dangerous and worrisome. In the diabetic patient in whom amputation is considered for infected or abscessed ulcers, however, sepsis is the rule rather than the exception. Local infection should not represent an impediment but attention must be paid to the preoperative management of cellulitis and bacterial infection. Systemic sepsis is a relative contraindication and should be controlled prior to surgery, except in cases in which infection cannot be stabilized without the amputation of the infection site.

Most diabetic wounds are infected with mixed flora. A culture that identifies the prominent pathologic microorganisms can facilitate antibiotic selection and, with appropriate antibiotic coverage, improve the chances for surgical success. For the elective procedure, prophylaxis against surgical infection should focus on those microorganisms suspected to be or continually present in the limb. The use of perioperative intravenous antibiotics is best started before surgery and continued through appropriate wound response in the postoperative period.

Wound closure with definitive amputation should never be performed in an attempt to gain control of advancing sepsis. The infection must be brought under control first, because the success of amputation surgery depends on adequate control of local ischemia and infection. Unless tissue is debrided aggressively, viable tissue can be further harmed because septic thrombosis then extends into otherwise normal tissue.

Any necrotizing process and active infection should be stabilized by surgical drainage, bed rest, elevation, warm compresses, and antibiotics. When possible, definitive surgery with wound closure should be delayed until the wound is no longer infected and the patient's general nutritional status has improved.

Following debridement, ulcers and gangrenous lesions are cultured, and broad-spectrum antibiotics are administered until the results of the culture and sensitivities are obtained. The nature of the infection does not have much prognostic value, provided the patient receives appropriate antibiotics. It is recommended that the patient be confined to strict bed rest with the limb elevated and warm compresses applied to the region. After cellulitis and the wet gangrenous process are under control, minimal secondary mechanical debridement may need to be performed in the operating room or at the bedside.

VASCULATURE CONSIDERATIONS

The final decision with respect to amputation is based on predictability of healing. Although many types of testing are relatively successful, the level of TCPO$_2$ represents the best predictor of healing. If levels are inadequate, vascular consultation should be considered. In considering the amputation of the second leg in a unilateral lower limb amputee, every diagnostic and surgical consideration should have the goal of preserving the maximum limb length to enhance function for the bilateral lower limb amputee. For example, if diagnostic tests will allow, a Syme ankle disarticulation on the contralateral side will benefit the previous transtibial amputee.

ANESTHESIA

General anesthesia may not be necessary for surgery in patients with diabetes. Even with a Syme ankle disarticulation, regional anesthesia can be sufficient. If pain control and muscle relaxation are needed for a more proximal amputation, the decision, with respect to technique, lies not so much with the procedure itself, but with the patient's cardiorespiratory status and concerns over systemic sepsis. It generally is unwise to violate the intrathecal space in the presence of systemic sepsis. Patients with diabetes also may have significant cardiorespiratory and renal problems that may be contraindications to general anesthesia. Because often these patients have a profound neuropathy, local or regional anesthesia works well. Infection occasionally may cause a well-localized tissue acidosis, which will inactivate, and thus prohibit, local anesthesia. Even under these conditions, however, regional anesthesia is successful and is preferred.

THE TOURNIQUET

There is no documented evidence that the routine use of a tourniquet during amputation surgery is associated with any more risk or complication than its use during other procedures. Its technical benefit in foot surgery, particularly in microvascular procedures, probably outweighs concern about increased risk of damage to fragile atherosclerotic vessels, aggravating neuropathy, or necrosis and infection. The decision is more properly based on surgical expedience, the need to have a clear indication of local vascularity versus the need to have enhanced visual capability, and reduced surgical time.

A tourniquet is generally not recommended during amputation surgery. Not using a tourniquet allows better visualization of the general perfusion of the foot, and also prevents the swelling that invariably occurs after the tourniquet has been deflated. Further, the metabolic changes that occur after the tourniquet has been removed can compromise an already tenuous limb. If a tourniquet must be used, it should be inflated after the limb is elevated and not by exsanguination of the foot and leg, particularly in the presence of infection. If ankle block anesthesia is feasible, an Esmarch bandage can be used as a supramalleolar tourniquet in cases with good blood flow.

SURGICAL TECHNIQUES

As much of the foot should be preserved as possible. In each case, however, the surgical procedure must be tailored to the limitations imposed by infection, deformity, and anticipated function. It is particularly advantageous, for example, to preserve length in the patient with intact circulation because in this subgroup of patients, abscess formation with wet gangrene predominates. Although ischemia may be present, the principal problem is infection. With early debridement and antibiotics, distal amputations may be feasible. In most older diabetics, however, gangrene is principally the result of ischemia. Instead of a florid infection, the gangrenous area is usually dry and associated with a necrotic process that has been present for some time. Successful revascularization often allows removal of the gangrenous part with reasonable assurance that the wound will heal.

The soft tissues are frequently atrophic such that incisions should be made carefully. Subcutaneous dissection should be minimal. Although all surgery is meticulously carried out, it may be accomplished without concern for precise anatomic landmarks. At no time should the skin or soft tissues be grasped with forceps. Skin hooks and rakes are used wherever possible and overzealous skin retraction is always avoided. Soft tissues and muscle are always gently retracted and protected. Bone cuts are made with sharp instruments, preferably using power equipment. All bone edges are carefully beveled and smoothed with a rongeur and a file or rasp. All infected gangrenous tissue must be radically debrided.

FOREFOOT AMPUTATIONS

Amputation of a toe through the base of the proximal phalanx is occasionally performed. However, the preferred level is the distal ray. Resection is carried out best through the neck of the metatarsal, preserving as much length as can be allowed, based on the necessities of adequate closure. The fifth is usually resected slightly more proximally, in order to avoid a pressure area laterally with shoe wear.

Individual lesser toes can be resected; however, it is generally not advisable to leave a single fifth toe or to leave a single toe between two toe amputations.

The "tennis racquet" incision is most frequently chosen. The skin ellipses are kept sufficiently long to allow tension from the closure. In diabetic patients, the metatarsal head is transected through the proximal portion of the incision, often just with a bone cutter or rongeur. Bone edges are then beveled and smoothed. The tendons are pulled distally and transected, such that a minimum of hypovascular tissue remains in the stump area.

With the first and fifth toe, a similar incision with a proximal portion based more to the side of the foot is used. Care is taken to avoid arterial supply, and again the flaps are left sufficiently long for tension-free closure. The metatarsal stump on the first ray is beveled medially and on the fifth ray beveled laterally, and smoothed to avoid subcutaneous pressure.

The preferred level of amputation in the forefoot is transmetatarsal if generalized necrosis and/or infection is present. Again, the level ide-

ally is just proximal to the metatarsal heads. Preferably, the skin incision is planned to allow a longer plantar flap, which offers more suitable protection to both the plantar surface and the osteotomized bone tips. Again, care is taken to bevel skin margins and tendons are retracted distally before division. At this level attention to skin closure must assure stability of the subcutaneous tissue and avoid dead space. This is best carried out in a combined skin subcutaneous single-layer closure, again with nonabsorbable suture and drain if necessary.

Drains

Drains should be routinely used if wounds and incisions are closed primarily. A polyethylene tube is placed subcutaneously through the dorsum of the foot into the wound. During wound closure, suction is placed on the catheter to maintain their patency. After the wound is completely closed, the catheter is irrigated with a continuous infusion of Ringer's lactate or normal saline. Antibiotic solutions are possibly hazardous and not necessary because the patient is receiving them intravenously. The irrigating fluid that exits between the sutures dilutes the bacteria and hematoma, simultaneously washing out debris.

Lisfranc and Chopart Level Disarticulations

An amputation at these levels may fail because equinus or equinovarus deformity may develop after surgery and is frequently followed by plantar-distal ulceration in insensate diabetics as described below. However, if the amputation is performed correctly, this complication almost never arises. The advantage of amputation at these levels is that the patient is not dependent on a prosthesis and is able to wear a regular shoe with an ankle-foot orthosis and a shoe filler.

Whenever possible, a Chopart (midtarsal) amputation is recommended over a Syme ankle disarticulation. The Chopart amputation is indicated when there is more extensive necrosis and gangrene of the forefoot, which precludes performing a transmetatarsal or Lisfranc amputation.

The problems of equinus or equinovarus contracture and deformity can be lessened to a large extent by carefully planned surgery. An Achilles tendon lengthening, most easily performed percutaneously, is essential in Chopart and often needed in transmetatarsal amputations. In some

FIGURE 20
Chopart disarticulation. **Left** and **Center,** Skin markings for a Chopart amputation. Lateral (left) and dorsal (center). **Right,** Following ablation of the forefoot, the articular surfaces of the talus and calcaneus are denuded.

(Reproduced with permission from Myerson M: Amputations of the midfoot and hindfoot, in Myerson M (ed): *Current Therapy in Foot and Ankle Surgery.* St. Louis, MO, Mosby-Year Book, 1993.)

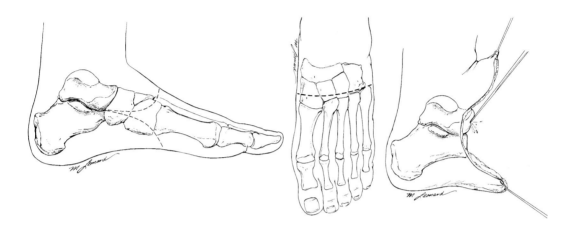

FIGURE 21
Left, Following the steps outlined in Figure 20, the skin flaps are checked to ensure closure without tension **(left)** and the anterior tibial tendon is pulled into the wound **(Center)** and secured to the lateral surface of the talus with staples

(Right). (Reproduced with permission from Myerson M: Amputations of the midfoot and hindfoot, in Myerson M (ed): *Current Therapy in Foot and Ankle Surgery.* St. Louis, MO, Mosby-Year Book, 1993.)

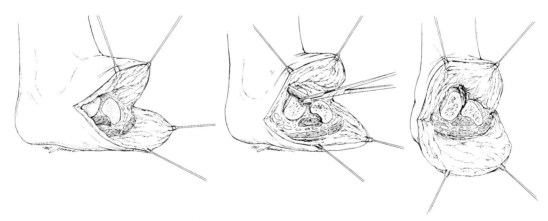

instances, a 1-inch strip of the Achilles tendon can be resected to prevent contracture following tenotomy. In addition, transfer of the extensor tendons and the anterior tibial tendon to the talus must be performed to prevent equinus deformity (Figs. 20 and 21).

Unlike the skin flap in a transmetatarsal amputation, a long plantar flap is not as important in midfoot amputations. A closure is recommended in which the plantar skin is just slightly longer than the dorsal skin; it is performed through a large fish-mouth incision. The plantar flap should join the dorsal skin at the weightbearing margins of the forefoot. Occasionally, the plantar flap is compromised because of necrosis, and the design for closure is modified so that even more of a dorsal flap closure is present.

Varus deformity is not usually a problem at this level because the posterior tibial tendon insertion has been sacrificed distally and the anterior tibial tendon will be reattached to the neck of the talus. However, varus may occur if the posterior tibial tendon becomes adherent to the plantar medial soft tissues, in which case, the tendon is cut or removed. The anterior tibial tendon can be sutured to the periosteal remnant at the neck of the talus or passed through a drill hole in the neck of the talus. Stapling is the easiest method of attachment of the tendon to the talar head at an area denuded of cartilage.

For the Lisfranc level, the foot is disarticulated at the tarsometatarsal joints. A short transmetatarsal amputation, however, is a better functional level because the attachments of the anterior tibial and peroneal tendons are more easily preserved. As much of the soft tissues around the amputation site as possible should be preserved, including the intrinsic muscles through subperiosteal dissection of the metatarsals. These local muscle pedicles can be of immense importance in the presence of inadequate flaps distally, and can provide extra bulk to the flap. When resecting the first and second metatarsals, the first dorsal and plantar interosseous muscles are carefully dissected out in order to preserve the dorsalis pedis and its perforating branch. These muscles can then be sutured loosely to the adjacent periosteum.

For Lisfranc amputations, the balance of the extrinsic tendons must be preserved. The posterior tibial tendon insertion is preserved at this level; if the peroneal attachments are lost, the foot tends to drift into varus with time. The anterior tibial and peroneus longus tendon insertions can be carefully preserved, because they both have a slip of insertion on the medial cuneiform. The peroneus brevis insertion also can be saved by preserving the base of the fifth metatarsal. With the loss of the function of the extrinsic toe extensors, the foot may also develop an equinus contracture, although not as severe as may occur after the Chopart amputation. Percutaneous fractional Achilles tendon

lengthening should be done. Another method of avoiding varus and equinus deformities is to carefully reattach the extensor and anterior tibial tendons to the dorsolateral aspect of the foot. Insertion into the lateral cuneiform is usually adequate.

Skin closure and postoperative irrigation are described above. The foot requires careful postoperative immobilization in dorsiflexion in a cast or with a carefully molded splint.

Pirogoff Amputation

While not generally applied as a primary level of amputation, the classic Pirogoff amputation can be used to salvage a planned Chopart when there is insufficient skin tissue for closure. The talus can be pulled forward, and the section carried around the body of the talus and into the subtalar joint. The talus is then delivered from the mortise and an osteotome is used to clear cartilage and subchondral bone from the plafond of the tibia. The distal end of the calcaneus at the calcaneocuboid joint is then osteotomized and rotated 90° into the plafond. Sufficient bone is removed to establish a firm position without undue tension on the skin flap (Fig. 22).

A percutaneous Achilles tendon lengthening is performed and all exposed tendons and collagenous tissue are debrided. Threaded pins or a long threaded screw are then passed percutaneously from the weightbearing surface, proximal into the tibia. A drain is then inserted and a bulky dressing or postoperative cast is applied. Jacobs recommends that sutures be left in for about 6 weeks, at which point the pins may be removed if radiographs show early callous bridging.[70] The disadvantages include waiting for bony or firm fibrous union and the lack of modern prosthetic components for this level, leading to a poor cosmetic result compared to the Syme level.

Calcanectomy

The surgical treatment of acute and chronic infections of the calcaneus presents considerable difficulty in the patient with diabetes. Calcaneal osteomyelitis in the diabetic patient is best treated with a total calcanectomy rather than repeated debridements, which usually fail. A plantar longitudinal incision is used, the ulcer is elliptically excised, and any infected tissue or

FIGURE 22
Pirogoff amputation. **Left,** Well-padded
weightbearing stump with leg length
nearly normal. **Right,** Radiograph.

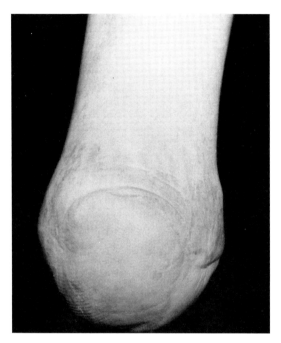
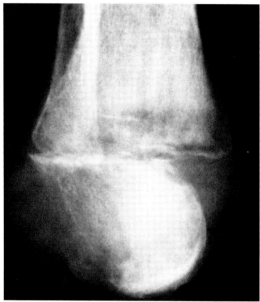

pus is evacuated from the deep fascial space. The insertion of the Achilles tendon, the talocalcaneal interosseous ligaments, and the capsules of the subtalar and calcaneocuboid joints are sectioned. It is important to remove all debris and potentially infective tissue. Closure of the subcutaneous tissue and skin is loose. These wounds tend to drain for a long period of time. A total contact cast can be applied as soon as the acute inflammatory phase has settled, even in the presence of continued drainage, but the cast must be changed more frequently under these circumstances. Patients finally ambulate with a polypropylene splint with a Plastazote and foam filler in the region of the heel defect.

The Syme Ankle Disarticulation

There are a number of factors that recommend the Syme ankle disarticulation; for example, the greater length of the leg makes rehabilitation and prosthetic wear far easier. With the final stages of maturation of the stump, the patient is able to walk short distances without a prosthesis in an emergency. Habitual walking without a prosthesis will lead to displacement of the heel pad.

Patients who are candidates for the Syme ankle disarticulation must be able to bear weight in a prosthesis; should have a heel pad that, ideally, is free of wounds; and should have a Doppler systolic pressure at the ankle at 70 mm Hg or more and an ischemic index that is greater than 0.45. It is especially important that these levels be present in the posterior tibial artery. The ankle and more proximal regions should be free of acute infection and intraoperative bleeding should occur in the skin of the flaps within 3 minutes after the tourniquet is released. A two-stage amputation is particularly indicated in cases in which there is extensive infection in the midfoot, whereas the more commonly performed single-stage amputation is indicated in cases of dry gangrene, chronic ulceration, or infection limited to the forefoot.

An incision is made directly anterior to the ankle joint, then carried medially and laterally to points approximately 1.5 cm distal to the malleoli (Fig. 23). From these points, the incision is carried distally from each malleolus in a stirrup configuration just distal to the heel pad. This incision is deepened without any dissection of subcutaneous tissue planes. The tendons are incised and allowed to retract. The posterior tibial neurovascular bundle, which lies immediately posteromedial, must be carefully preserved, because the posterior tibial artery supplies the entire flap. The Achilles tendon attachment is carefully divided from the calcaneus without perforating the skin (Fig. 23). It is important to dissect out the calcaneus in a plane beneath the periosteum in order that the fascial septae of the heel pad are preserved to provide shock absorption during gait. No attempt is made to trim any redundant skin at the corners of the flaps because to do so may jeopardize their blood supply. The malleoli are cut flush with the tibial plafond and also narrowed with an ostetome. The plantar fascia of the heel pad is sutured to three drill holes in the anterior tibia to provide excellent stability. The skin is closed with nonabsorbable sutures without any tension. A closed continuous irrigation drain is fashioned from a Foley catheter or Shirley drain. One liter of normal saline is used every 8 hours. The wound is usually stable enough for the patient to commence walking in a well-padded cast at about 4 weeks.

If a two-stage procedure has been necessary, the second stage is performed after about 6 weeks (Fig. 24). Medial and lateral incisions are made directly over the dog ears, and the malleoli are osteotomized flush with the ankle joint, leaving the articular cartilage intact. The malleoli are also narrowed with an osteotome.

AMPUTATION CLOSURE

All incisions are closed loosely with absolutely no tension using 2-0 or 3-0 nylon sutures for skin only. Subcutaneous sutures are not used. This loose approximation of the wound prevents necrosis of the wound edges, which are marginally ischemic. If the incision cannot be com-

pletely closed without tension, it is preferable either to leave the wound open and allow secondary healing by granulation or to cover the wound with split-thickness skin grafts. These grafts can be obtained with a dermatome from the amputated part and meshed for immediate application or obtained as pinch grafts at a later stage. Pinch grafts may stimulate the further formation of adjacent granulations, which in turn can be covered with additional grafts, thus speeding up closure. If there is insufficient skin for definitive and complete coverage, the foot should not be shortened further by bone resection unless the defect is large. In general it is best to avoid split grafts directly on the distal or plantar surfaces of the partial foot because these tend to ulcerate with walking. Dorsal wounds may be left open and later covered with split-thickness skin grafts. This does not work on the plantar surface of the foot, however, especially in weightbearing areas. If a guillotine amputation has been performed for severe sepsis, the wound is either left open to granulate or excised and closed secondarily at 10 to 14 days.

POSTOPERATIVE CARE

It is important to place the limb in a protected position after surgery. Patients are encouraged to keep the limb elevated for approximately 3 weeks after surgery. Diabetic wounds take a long time to heal, and it is advisable to leave sutures in place for about 3 or 4 weeks in most cases. Systemic antibiotics are continued after surgery until wounds are healed. There are no absolute criteria regarding the use of postoperative antibiotics and they should be prescribed on an individual basis depending on the appearance of the wound. Intravenous antibiotics are recommended for approximately 10 days after surgery, followed by oral antibiotics as required.

Depending on the type and closure of the amputation, once the wounds begin to heal, the patient may commence partial weightbearing. The recognized benefits of immediate casting, commonplace for leg amputations, present the same physiologic advantage to diabetic foot amputation surgery. The concept is enhanced when considered as a continuation of occlusive casting. The theoretical concern over occult compartment syndrome is greatly outweighed by the

FIGURE 23
Syme disarticulation, first-stage procedure. **Top left,** Surface markings for a Syme amputation. **Bottom left,** The talus is dissected free from its ligamentous attachments. **Bottom center,** The calcaneus is removed by careful subperiosteal dissection. **Bottom right,** The skin is apposed loosely. (Reproduced with permission from Myerson M: Amputations of the midfoot and hindfoot, in Myerson M (ed): *Current Therapy in Foot and Ankle Surgery.* St. Louis, MO, Mosby-Year Book, 1993.)

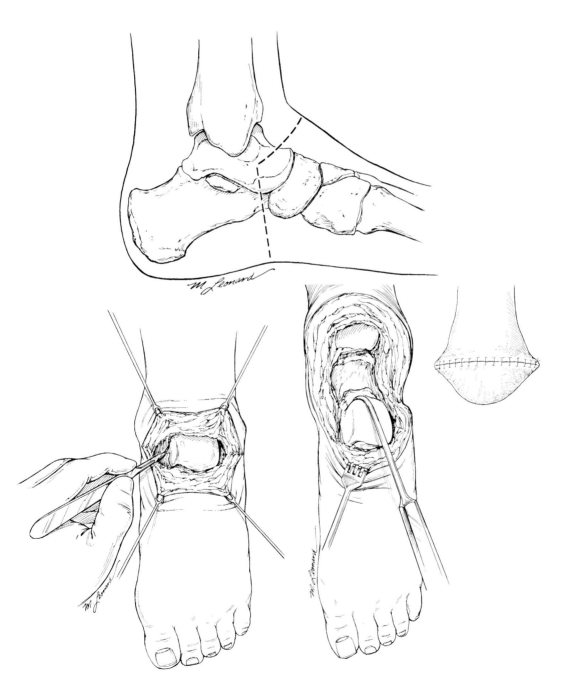

FIGURE 24
The Syme's second-stage procedure is performed through elliptical medial and lateral incisions. (Reproduced with permission from Myerson M: Amputations of the midfoot and hindfoot, in Myerson M (ed): *Current Therapy in Foot and Ankle Surgery.* St. Louis, MO, Mosby-Year Book, 1993.)

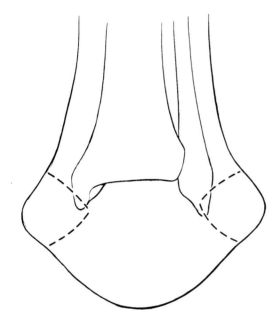

recognized advantages allowed by the carefully applied cast; eg, control of edema, hemostasis, soft-tissue immobilization, prevention of skin-flap motion and protection of the wound from trauma. The amputation level should have been sufficient enough to alleviate the need for any specialized wound care; thus, the cast dressing can greatly simplify postoperative care.

Nonweightbearing casts are used for 2 weeks. The initial cast is changed after 4 to 7 days, and the wound is inspected. After the second week, a well-fitted total contact cast is applied and the patient begins ambulation. Some patients require crutches or other ambulatory assistance until quite independent, but most patients can support full weightbearing after a few days in this walking cast. Use of the cast is discontinued as soon as the wound has matured.

The use of the total contact cast immensely improves the postoperative management of these patients. It helps mobilize the patient rapidly, thereby avoiding many of the problems associated with prolonged bed rest. The presence of edema, local increases in temperature, and tenuous wound edges are all indications for continuing total contact cast treatment.

Lisfranc amputation stumps are usually long enough to suspend a shoe, but because of the tendency to develop an equinus deformity, can make shoe fitting difficult. Pressure on the plantar aspect of the distal foot can be prevented by stabilizing the ankle with a polypropylene ankle-foot orthosis but Achilles tendon lengthening is often preferable. Chopart amputations are too short to suspend a shoe. These patients may also be fitted with an ankle-foot orthosis or with a more cosmetic custom-molded partial foot prosthesis from which the shoe is suspended. The only drawback to the Syme ankle disarticulation is its somewhat bulbous stump. The prosthesis must be similarly large to accommodate the stump, making it less attractive for use in females. Most women have smaller feet, however, making the disparity much less than in men, especially with newer prosthetic designs.

SHOE MODIFICATIONS FOR PARTIAL FOOT AMPUTATION

Objectives

Provide a Shoe Filler The shoe filler provided for the amputated portion of the forefoot will help prevent creasing of the shoe at the point of the amputation, avoiding both skin breakdown and eventual collapse of the shoe. The addition of a steel shank and rocker sole will greatly assist in function. A filler also helps control the remaining foot inside the shoe, decreasing shear. The use of a filler can eliminate the need for more costly, less cosmetically appealing custom-made shoes. In most cases, the filler can be incorporated into the diabetic patient's insert (Fig. 13, *left*).[71]

Equalize Weightbearing Amputation of a portion of the foot will often result in altered patterns of weightbearing in the remaining part of the foot. Just as with any diabetic foot, any areas of excessive pressure must be eliminated and even distribution of weightbearing maintained.

Protect and Accommodate the Remaining Portion of the Foot Because the presence of an amputation implies severe foot problems, special care must be taken to protect and accommodate the remaining portion of the foot at risk. Skin grafts, scar tissue, or other postsurgical complications must also be taken into consideration when providing prescription footwear for a foot that has undergone partial amputation.

Improve Gait When part of the foot has been amputated, a natural gait pattern is no longer possible on the unshod foot. The addition of an appropriate type of rocker sole can often improve the gait pattern after an amputation.

Shoes

A shoe with a blucher opening and a long medial counter will best control the remaining foot and help decrease shear. The upper should be made of a soft, moldable leather to accommodate and protect the remaining foot. Custom-made shoes are generally not necessary with a transmetatarsal amputation because with the aid of a filler, enough of the foot remains to keep a shoe on; however, a shoe with a shortened toe box may be considered if the patient finds it cosmetically acceptable.

External Shoe Modifications

An extended steel shank in conjunction with an appropriate rocker sole can reduce pressure and impact shock, while aiding propulsion and reducing the amount of shoe distortion. The use of a cushion heel will further minimize impact shock. Medial and/or lateral flares may be added to stabilize and control the amputated foot and decrease shear.

Orthoses

A total contact insole with a filler will help to stabilize or restrict joint motion, accommodate bony prominences and deformities, decrease shear and shoe distortion, and equalize weight-bearing. A sock designed for transmetatarsal amputations also may be helpful in protecting and accommodating the remaining foot.

DIABETIC NEUROARTHROPATHY

The destruction of joints in patients with sensory loss from syphilis was described by Charcot in the last century.

Now, neuroarthropathy (the Charcot joints) of the foot and ankle in the patient with diabetes mellitus is a common orthopaedic problem, the outcome of which depends on proper management. The incidence of neuroarthropathy in diabetes ranges from 1% to 2.5%. Neuroarthropathy occurs most commonly in the midfoot and hindfoot. As noted, a clear correlation between the level of diabetic control and the onset of progression has been demonstrated; thus, most patients are on average 40 years old at presentation. Because the life span of diabetic patients continues to increase, many orthopaedic surgeons will have an opportunity to manage this problem.

The (neuroarthropathic) Charcot foot in the patient with diabetes is common and can ultimately lead to amputation. Although other elements of neuropathy and ischemia are often present, they may be addressed to some extent by revascularization without resorting to amputation (Fig. 1). It is generally thought that the pathologic process represents an acceleration of osteoarthritis that is precipitated by trauma in the neuropathic joint.[72] Structural breakdown of the foot (which leads to wound problems) and osteomyelitis are far more difficult to treat.

CONCEPTS OF TREATMENT

The treatment of the Charcot foot and ankle is influenced by the stage of arthropathy. Eichenholtz[73] described three stages of development of the Charcot joint that are fairly typical of the course of events from the initial phase of the arthropathy through healing. In stage 1, which is characterized by acute inflammation associated with hyperemia and erythema, the bone dissolves and fragmentation and dislocations are common. In stage 2, which is characterized by bony coalescence and decreased swelling, there is radiographic evidence of periosteal new bone formation, even when the initial injury was a joint dislocation rather than fracture. In stage 3, bony consolidation and healing occurs.

The initial diagnosis of acute neuroarthropathy is relatively straightforward, based on painless swelling associated with warmth of the affected area. Although radiographs are helpful, the typical changes of neuroarthropathy, such as fragmentation and periosteal new bone formation, are not often present during this acute stage. This can lead to aspiration attempts and even prolonged antibiotic treatment when misdiagnosed as osteomyelitis.

Treatment approaches for neuroarthropathy have changed significantly since the mid 1980s. The goal of any treatment program for the Charcot foot is to achieve a plantigrade weightbearing surface that is free of infection. In addition to these parameters, the foot and ankle must be stable and at least braceable. Whether the phase is acute or chronic and involves the midfoot, hindfoot, or ankle, most forms of Charcot breakdown are treated nonsurgically. The accepted treatment for neuropathic arthropathy of the foot and ankle has been prolonged immobilization in a brace or plaster cast until there is radiographic evidence of consolidation, and clinical stability of the foot and ankle has been restored. These methods of treatment are effective in most patients, particularly when promptly instituted. Severe deformity, however, may develop despite appropriate immobilization and protected weightbearing. Immobilization of the limb does not guarantee additional deformity will not occur.

Although some reports indicate deformity may progress in the immobilized limb even if it is not subjected to weightbearing, others have experienced different results.[74] Deformity may indeed worsen in a cast, but patients with these conditions do bear weight on the limb, due to a combination of any of a number of factors—neuropathy, noncompliance, or inability to use crutches or a walker because of problems with proprioception and balance. One question is whether a long leg cast with the knee flexed would achieve a more reliable end result under these circumstances.

The mainstay of treatment for neuropathic arthropathy, once diagnosed, continues to be prolonged external immobilization in a plaster cast or orthosis.[74] An orthosis is the traditional method of managing chronic deformity of the hindfoot and ankle. This orthosis may be any of a number of types: a vertical double upright ankle-foot orthosis (AFO) attached to a shoe, a molded polypropylene posterior AFO, or a clamshell type. The patellar tendon bearing (PTB) orthosis has recently been evaluated by Saltzman and associates,[75] who assessed the effect of shoe wear, custom-made inserts, PTB orthoses, and extra-padded PTB orthoses on load transmission

to neuroarthropathic feet. They found that a properly fitted PTB orthosis can reduce load transmission to the Charcot foot, but in a reliable manner only to the hindfoot. Adding extra padding to the orthosis further decreased the mean peak force by 32%. They recommended that a PTB orthosis not be used to reduce vertical load transmission to the midfoot or forefoot. For long-term use, the PTB orthosis should be used for treatment of hindfoot disorders only and adjusted regularly to ensure adequate fit.

Deformity of the hindfoot and ankle, however, may not be amenable to bracing, because these structures are far too unstable to be maintained in adequate alignment by either an orthosis or a cast. The stresses of weightbearing in patients with deformity may preclude the possibility of bracing. To avoid the complications of unstable neuroarthropathy, surgical treatment is occasionally warranted, particularly when consolidation and healing of the neuropathic fracture and dislocation have not taken place. With either a varus or valgus deformity of the hindfoot or ankle, it is particularly difficult to keep the foot in a plantigrade position centered under the leg. Although a Syme ankle disarticulation or a transtibial amputation eliminates the immediate problem, many amputees experience limitations in day-to-day functional activities, necessitating a significant modification in life-style. Amputees have an increased energy requirement, frequently have limited cardiac reserve, are often overweight, and have a marked risk for future contralateral amputation. For these reasons, attempts at limb salvage are recommended wherever possible.

Although surgical treatment for neuropathic arthropathy of the foot and ankle is an option, under most circumstances, this should not be the initial treatment of choice. Myerson and associates reported that at an average of approximately 4 years after arthrodesis, salvage proved to be successful in 93% of patients with intractable diabetic neuropathic arthropathy of the hindfoot and ankle treated with open reduction and arthrodesis.[76,77] Certainly, surgical treatment must be considered part of the armamentarium for managing the deformed diabetic foot. This treatment program, however, was complex; 20 complications were encountered in 19 of the 29 patients. Enthusiasm for surgical treatment, therefore, must be tempered by the potential for complications during a difficult salvage procedure.

Other authors have reported on the results of surgical treatment of neuropathic arthropathy. Shibata and associates reported on results of extended hindfoot fusions in patients with leprotic neuropathic deformity.[78] They used an intramedullary nail for fixation. A solid arthrodesis occurred in 19 of the 26 patients. Stuart and Morrey[79] have reported on the results of ankle and hindfoot arthrodesis in 13 patients with insulin-dependent diabetes. Their results were satisfactory in only five of 13 patients. Complications developed in seven of the nine patients who showed radiographic signs of new neuroarthropathy. One of the problems that may have led to the high rate of failure in their patient group was that external fixation was used in nine of the 13 patients. External fixation is far from the ideal form of stabilization for these deformities, because it greatly increases the risk of infection.

Healing, from the acute inflammatory phase through coalescence and ultimate consolidation, takes a long period of time. Healing of the tarsometatarsal joint and midfoot takes approximately 6 to 12 months; healing of the hindfoot and ankle takes 12 to 24 months. The mainstay of treatment for most feet is adequate stabilization during this period of time to allow the tissues to heal and ultimately consolidate. Although deformity leading to recurrent ulceration may require surgery for claw toes, metatarsal head resections, and exostectomy, intervention with open reduction and arthrodesis is less commonly required. We (GS, SC) believe that it is important to recognize that open reduction alone is not sufficient to stabilize these joints.

Ideally, surgery should not be performed in the presence of an open wound. Therefore, if feasible, wounds are first healed with either a total contact cast or a split-thickness skin graft. If surgery is performed in the presence of an open wound, the infection rate is increased. Therefore, in the presence of an open wound with or without osteomyelitis, reconstruction and salvage must be staged. This problem exists, for example, over the malleoli, where ulceration may be associated with deeper infection. In these instances, it is preferable to debride the wound and bone and initiate treatment for osteomyelitis.

MIDFOOT DIABETIC NEUROARTHROPATHY

The treatment goal for patients with neuroarthropathy of the midfoot is to obtain a durable plantigrade foot for ambulation. Amputation remains a necessary management option in cases of infection or ischemia. By controlling the rate and severity of ulceration, however, a carefully designed treatment protocol can decrease the frequency with which amputations are required.

To initiate appropriate treatment, it is important to identify the stage of neuroarthropathy. Once immobilization and rest bring active neuroarthropathy under control, a brace or a total contact cast becomes the mainstay of treatment. The technique is well described and the benefits of this treatment for neuropathic ulceration have been recently reported.[36] Based on this study, the overall use of the total contact cast is effective in 75% of cases of neuroarthropathy involving the midfoot.

Although nonsurgical treatment measures are frequently successful, one group of eight acute fracture-dislocations of the tarsometatarsal joint may require surgery if significant dislocation is present, particularly if impending skin necrosis is present.[76] Open reduction and arthrodesis is warranted to prevent the complication of skin necrosis or ulceration. Because the disease process is acute, the bone density is usually adequate for fixation. Surgery should not be attempted if preoperative radiographs show evidence of bone resorption and fragmentation, because adequate screw purchase cannot be secured.[80]

Except for the treatment of infection, surgery should be avoided in the subacute stage of neuroarthropathy. Instead, nonsurgical means are used to carry the patient into the final stage of the process, at which point the signs of neuropathic activity have dissipated and bony coalescence has occurred. Rigid deformity of the midfoot is then more easily treated with molded accommodative orthoses. If the midfoot is unstable or severely deformed, then a Plastizote-lined polypropylene ankle-foot orthosis can be used. This provides total contact support, allowing the distribution of weightbearing forces away from plantar bony prominence. These bracing methods have proven effective in 75% of our patients.[76,80]

Based on results to date, it is believed that surgical salvage of the chronically deformed foot with exostectomy or realignment arthrodesis is a reasonable and appropriate alternative to amputation, if performed on appropriately selected patients. If amputation is required, a partial foot amputation maximizes independent function.[17,28] For patients with a systemic disease, such as diabetes, the difference between an ankle-foot orthosis with a shoe filler and a transtibial prosthesis is significant.

As noted by Sinha and associates,[81] joints adjacent to those with neuroarthropathic involvement can become activated by the disease process, probably because of altered biomechanical forces. There are seven examples of this in the series, all of which show distal to proximal reactivation. Limited ankle motion may play a role in reactivation and has been noted in 90% of patients with lower limb complications of diabetes.

The relationship of end-stage diabetic nephropathy and the need for salvage amputation is notable. Five of the seven patients who underwent amputation were treated for diabetic nephropathy. Amputation was required in all five to treat deep infection. Three of the five patients in this group were on immunosuppressive agents after renal transplantation. Of the entire series, these patients were undoubtedly the most difficult to manage successfully. Amputation, however, should not be construed as a failure of treatment, particularly if a partial foot amputation is performed.

The definition of stability, for the purpose of follow-up assessment, is based on an appreciation of the lifelong care that these feet require. Certainly, none of the feet considered stable at follow-up should have evidence of infection. Episodic swelling without warmth that resolves within a few weeks is not thought to represent active neuroarthropathy. Feet with no more than grade 1 ulceration that responds to a short-term total contact cast are stable as long as the ulcers are infrequent enough that surgery is not necessary. These patients are expected to return frequently for brace or insert adjustments because all of them, including those with a successful arthrodesis, require some form of orthotic shoe support. The goal of treatment is to obtain a stable and plantigrade foot and to avoid amputation wherever possible.

Acute Midfoot Neuroarthropathy

For *acute* neuroarthropathy, the mainstay of treatment is to rest the limb, restrict ambulation and activities, and immobilize the region with a cast. The indication for surgery in this acute setting is very specific, surgery should be performed only for a severe *dislocation* that is unstable and manually reducible. Any bone fragmentation or periosteal new bone formation is a contraindication to surgery. Open reduction and arthrodesis is indicated in these patients to prevent skin necrosis and acute ulceration after reduction of edema. Because the disease process is acute, the bone density is usually adequate for fixation. Surgery should not be attempted if preoperative radiographs show evidence of bone absorption and fragmentation, because profound osteopenia may be present, precluding stable reduction and fixation.

Surgery should be delayed until after swelling has resolved, because swelling increases problems with wound closure and likelihood of infection. This swelling has to be monitored very closely because the displaced tarsal and metatarsal bones will often cause skin necrosis. The AVI foot pump (Kendall, Mansfield, MA) can be used to reduce edema in the foot. The foot pump has been used successfully in the presence of neuropathic swelling of the foot. Edema should be monitored closely to prevent pressure and ischemic necrosis of prominent parts of the foot. Between 4 and 6 hours of intermittent compression is often sufficient to decrease all edema in the foot and prepare the foot for surgery. Prophylactic cephalosporin antibiotics are used routinely.

A tourniquet is not recommended and surgery is performed using regional ankle block anesthesia. Because arthrodesis is the procedure of choice, bone graft is occasionally required for *acute* neuroarthropathy, but its use depends on the magnitude of the deformity. In the event of significant bone loss, iliac crest bone should be used, but it may be possible to harvest smaller quantities of graft from the calcaneus. Grafting is usually unnecessary in the setting of acute fracture dislocation, because minimal bone resorption and destruction have occurred. Bone graft is invariably required for reconstruction of chronic neuroarthropathy.

SURGICAL TECHNIQUE

The incisions are planned according to the pattern of dislocation, the most common of which is disruption of the medial column involving the first metatarsal and medial cuneiform. Here, a single dorsal incision is made medial to the extensor hallucis longus tendon. In patients with middle column disruption involving the second and third metatarsocuneiform joints, two incisions are made—a long incision centered over the space between the second and third metatarsals and a smaller incision placed medially over the first metatarsal and medial cuneiform. Thick skin flaps are raised without much attention paid to superficial nerves.

Fibrous scar and granulation tissue should be removed from the joint spaces. Thin flexible chisels or fine sharp osteotomes are used to denude the articular surfaces. Manual reduction is performed and temporary internal fixation is obtained using 0.062-inch Kirschner wires or the guide pins for cannulated screws. It is important to obtain intraoperative anteroposterior and lateral radiographs to assess the reduction. Although fluoroscopic imaging is useful to guide the insertion of the pins, it is not sufficient to determine alignment. The dislocation usually can be reduced by a maneuver that involves grasping the hallux and pulling it into varus while simultaneously pushing with the thumb against the base of the first metatarsal and medial cuneiform. If this does not reduce the medial cuneiform, reduction can be accomplished using a small periosteal elevator. The base of the second metatarsal is the key to an anatomic reduction. Although achieving a precise reduction and alignment of the midfoot is not as important as for the patient without neuropathy, it is still preferable to restore a medial longitudinal arch and prevent recurrent pressure on the medial foot. Therefore, the use of compression screws for fixation is preferable to reduce the medial cuneiform directly into the second metatarsal and vice versa. The first screw is introduced medially from the medial cuneiform into the middle and lateral cuneiforms or the second metatarsal, depending on the pattern of dislocation. If the second metatarsal is laterally displaced, the screw can be directed obliquely and distally from the medial cuneiform into the second metatarsal base.

Subacute Midfoot Neuroarthropathy

It is important to distinguish between subacute and chronic neuroarthropathy of the midfoot. Although many feet become deformed, if the chronic stage is reached, the midfoot is by definition stable and stiff, but subacute arthropathy implies a midfoot, which although no longer swollen and inflamed, is nonetheless unstable. These feet are generally easy to protect in an extra depth shoe with a molded orthosis, and it is unlikely that patients with true chronic neuroarthropathy will require a midfoot arthrodesis. Some feet remain in a subacute phase permanently, the midfoot is deformed and unstable, and a "spongy" fibrous arthrosis is present at the apex of the deformity. A rocker bottom deformity is present, with an apex medial or lateral, depending on which bones are prominent on the plantar surface of the foot. In these feet, sagittal plane motion occurs through this pseudoarthrosis, and the hindfoot remains fixed in equinus. The rockerbottom deformity is always associated with a fixed hindfoot equinus. The posterior soft tissues, including the Achilles and flexor tendons, are contracted. In addition to midfoot arthrodesis, an Achilles tendon lengthening is integral to the treatment of this deformity. The remaining long flexor tendons rarely require lengthening. The magnitude of this equinus contracture is best evaluated on a weight-bearing lateral radiograph of the foot. The lateral radiograph will show that the forefoot must be redirected (plantarflexed) in line with the hindfoot, which must be corrected through posterior soft-tissue releases.

Chronic Midfoot Neuroarthropathy

The need for arthrodesis of the midfoot in the setting of chronic neuroarthropathy is less common. Most feet can be successfully treated with accommodative orthoses in a wide, extra-depth shoe with a rockerbottom sole. If this type of shoe is unsatisfactory, a custom-molded shoe with a steel shank and a molded AFO can be used. Unlike the unstable foot found in subacute neuroarthropathy, these feet are stiff and generally stable, so that the deformity usually can be protected with the appropriate shoe. If ulceration recurs over a long bone prominence, tarsal ostectomy is an alternative form of treatment. Unlike the hindfoot and ankle, ostectomy of the midfoot is a good option and should be considered if ulceration recurs. Ostectomy works best when the arthropathy is chronic, the deformity is rigid and stable, and no pseudoarthrosis or false motion occurs across the site of the original fracture dislocation process. Therefore, this chronic but stable deformity is generally easier to treat because the foot can be fitted with an appropriate accommodative shoe and orthosis. If ulceration recurs despite this treatment program, ostectomy is indicated and the offending bone is shaved down or removed. This may involve the cuneiform, cuboid, navicular, or a combination of these bones.

OSTECTOMY

The apex of midfoot collapse is often the cuboid fourth metatarsal articulation, and even when the bony prominence beneath the midfoot ulcer is more medial, third cuneiform articulation, the lateral approach is preferred. A transverse incision is placed below the peroneus brevis proximal fifth metatarsal base. Dissection is carried deep to the plantar fascia along digiti brevis, along the osseous course of the peroneus longus. The neurovascular structures are then safely protected by the quadratus planti and second- and third-layer soft tissues.

The offending bony prominence will be palpated directly "beneath" the area of ulceration. A sharp osteotome and rongeurs can then be employed to achieve a flattened surface. The amount of bone necessary to achieve this is removed. The surrounding osseous tissue is smoothed with rasp and rongeur, and the wound loosely approximated with nonabsorbable suture.

The editor's technique is to perform the surgical dissection through an impregnated barrier drape to prevent contamination from the chronic area of ulceration. Then, following skin closure, a xeroform dressing is placed over the skin incision. The barrier drape is then removed from the ulcer and careful debridement to viable dermal tissue carried out. The ulcer is similarly dressed, and a plaster cast reinforced with fiberglass and covered for skin protection is applied.

Patients with stable chronic neuroarthropathy rarely have pain, although it may occur when the forefoot is severely abducted, the midfoot is severely pronated, and the hindfoot is in equinus.

Combined Midfoot Arthrodesis

Prior to the midfoot approach, soft-tissue lengthening is performed posteriorly with percu-taneous triple hemisection technique for the Achilles tendon. A stab incision is made centrally in the posterior aspect of the Achilles tendon and then directed subcutaneously. The incisions on the tendon are spaced approximately three quarters of an inch apart. The Achilles tendon should be lengthened before work is begun on the midfoot, because no effective dorsiflexion lever on the foot is present once the midfoot is open. If the hindfoot is still in equinus following Achilles tendon lengthening, the other long flexor tendons may require lengthening. In severe rockerbottom deformity, these tendons would have to be approached through a lateral incision over the peroneal tendons and a posteromedial incision posterior to the medial malleolus.

Three longitudinal incisions are typically used to reconstruct these feet: dorsomedial, central, and lateral. I (GJS) recommend a transverse incision across the midfoot with the advantage of improved exposure. Transection of superficial nerves is not important, however, this incision disrupts the superficial veins and potentially could cause problems with wound healing.

Thick skin flaps are raised regardless of the method of these incisions. The dislocated joints are approached by resecting the fibrous scar. Although an osteotome may be used to perform these plantar cuts, a small microsagittal saw blade may be preferable. The extruded bone fragments on the plantar surfaces must be removed and are usually accessible through the dorsal incisions. A laminar spreader is placed into the wound between the tarsal and metatarsal bones and placed on distraction, and the bone fragments on the plantar surface are removed with a rongeur.

Once the bone fragments, debris, and fibrous tissue have been removed, the forefoot is reduced to the midfoot by adduction and plantarflexion. Large gaps are usually present between the tarsal and metatarsal bones. Approximation of the bone ends should not be attempted at this time. Temporary internal fixation with Kirschner wires is used and anteroposterior and lateral radiographs are obtained. After the intraoperative radiographs are obtained, permanent fixation and final correction are planned. Bone graft is usually necessary. The bone graft is morcellized and only cancellous bone fragments (2 × 3 mm) are used.

Permanent fixation of the midfoot is not easy because of osteopenia and the irregular size and shapes of the remaining bones and joints. Although the insertion of crossed pins from the first and fifth metatarsals is relatively easy, this fixation construct is not very stable and compression lag screws may be preferred. One screw that is always helpful in these chronic midfoot reconstructions is a 6.5- or 7.0-mm lag screw introduced from the medial cuneiform transversely across the foot into the cuboid. The other screws are introduced from the medial and lateral aspects of the foot obliquely. Cannulated screws are much easier to insert because the guide pins can be introduced and radiographs obtained before the screws are inserted. Occasionally *threaded* Steinmann pins are needed because of the orientation and quality of the bones. Threaded pins are preferable because they cause less motion at the skin interface and are therefore less likely to be associated with pin-tract infections. These are left in place for approximately 3 months and should be used cautiously because they protrude from the skin during that time.

HINDFOOT AND ANKLE DEFORMITY

Regardless of the magnitude of the varus or valgus deformity, bracing usually succeeds if the ankle and subtalar joint are stable. If the foot can be maintained under the axis of the leg during the acute or subacute phases of neuroarthropathy, despite bone dissolution or destruction, the foot will usually be stable. This, of course, requires prolonged immobilization until the consolidation phase has been reached. This contrasts with the foot where gross dislocation of the tarsus or ankle is present, which may occur during either the acute or chronic phases of neuroarthropathy. In the hindfoot, surgery should be performed only after the chronic phase is reached. The bone fragments are osteopenic during the acute hyperemic stage and adequate rigid internal fixation is not usually possible. Some feet, however, may not reach a chronic phase of bony consolidation. Dislocation or subluxation persists and, in these feet, reconstruction is performed during the subacute stage of arthropathy.

Arthrodesis is therefore indicated in the hindfoot and ankle only when the severely unstable joint is not amenable to bracing, or in those patients for whom bracing has been attempted but who have repeated ulceration. Surgery is also occasionally indicated during the acute phase of hindfoot neuroarthropathy when there is an acute fracture or dislocation followed by disorderly fragmentation and loss of alignment. An acute fracture-dislocation of the ankle that is amenable to open reduction and internal fixation should be treated in a patient with diabetes in the same manner as in a patient without neuropathy. Diabetes is not a contraindication to internal fixation of acute fractures of the ankle. In fact, even more caution should be exercised to ensure that the fracture heals uneventfully. Unless these fractures are immobilized postoperatively for a long period of time, malunion and fragmentation of the talus may occur. Immobilization below the knee that sacrifices full range of motion should be considered in these patients until there is complete healing with no signs of warmth or swelling. The patient should not bear weight for 3 months, and cast immobilization is continued for an additional 3 to 4 months until warmth and swelling have dissipated. Despite this caution, deformity may occur very rapidly in patients with neuropathy, and an early arthrodesis should be considered before inevitable ulceration and infection occur.

The same principles apply to an acute dislocation of the hindfoot and tarsal joints in which anticipated deformity is ultimately going to be difficult to brace. An example of this situation may be found in a patient with acute neuropathic dislocation of the naviculum with considerable deformity. The alternative for treatment in this patient would be to follow the course of neuroarthropathy with limb elevation, immobilization, and bracing in the hope of avoiding eventual ulceration. With this deformity, however, it is highly likely that ulceration will occur due to the prominence of the naviculum on the plantar medial aspect of the foot. Salvage could be performed later with excision of the naviculum or a later arthrodesis. However, it is likely that with time, the deformity will increase, which may be difficult to salvage subsequently. Early surgery therefore may be indicated.

As in the midfoot, it is preferable to avoid surgery on the hindfoot and ankle in the presence of an open wound. This is not always easy because the nature of the instability causing as well as perpetuating the wound may preclude the possibility of spontaneous wound healing. In these patients, strict bed rest and a split-thickness skin graft may be used to obtain coverage followed by reconstructive surgery as soon as it is feasible before breakdown again occurs. If the hindfoot is grossly unstable, or if osteomyelitis is present, an external fixator may be used to achieve temporary stability. After the wound inflammation has subsided, skin coverage is obtained followed by arthrodesis. Osteomyelitis is treated aggressively with debridement and appropriate antibiotics, and the definitive surgery is delayed until it is the osteomyelitis is completely resolved. External fixation should not be used routinely to secure immobilization because of the markedly increased risk of infection. External fixation should be used only in the presence of focal sepsis that cannot be managed by other means. Rigid internal fixation with large cannulated 6.5- or 7.0-mm cancellous screws is preferred for the hindfoot and ankle.

Prophylactic intravenous antibiotics and a pneumatic tourniquet should be used for the hindfoot and ankle. A standard approach for a triple arthrodesis is used with a lateral incision dorsal to the peroneal tendons and a second dorsomedial incision medial to the anterior tibial tendon. A transfibular lateral approach is used for all tibiotalar fusions and is extended distally toward the sinus tarsi if a tibiotalocalcaneal or pantalar fusion is performed. A small medial incision is used to debride the talonavicular joint when it is included in the fusion. If needed, it can be used to explore the medial ankle and resect the medial malleolus, skin flaps should be minimal with soft-tissue attachment preserved wherever possible. Congruent surfaces are fashioned in the ankle and hindfoot to allow good bony contact and maximum inherent stability.

A talectomy and tibiocalcaneal fusion are performed if the talus is fragmented and avascular. If a talectomy is to be performed, supplemental bone graft should be used. Because of the plantar inclination of the posterior facet, the calcaneus cannot be apposed directly to the tibial plafond. If this is attempted, the hindfoot and calcaneus dorsiflex into a calcaneus position. Instead, a triangular-shaped bone graft needs to be inserted into the space created by resection of the joint surfaces. The graft can be fashioned using a strut of the fibula, a femoral head allograft, or trapezoidal pieces of tricortical bone from the iliac crest. This is augmented with copious cancellous bone chips. One way to obtain copious cancellous bone is to use a morsellized fibula graft by grinding down the fibula using a small acetabular reamer.

Determining the final position in which the foot is to be fused is one of the more difficult problems. This is particularly a problem following talectomy. The height of the foot is decreased and the soft-tissue bulk on the medial and lateral ankle obscures and distorts the alignment. For this reason, the limb should be draped proximal to the knee joint to allow full visualization of the foot and knee before definitive fixation. The foot is positioned plantigrade with the ankle in neutral dorsiflexion, 5° of hindfoot valgus, and slight external rotation. While slight valgus malunion is tolerated by the patient with neuropathy, varus deformity, however mild, will lead to ulceration along the lateral border of the foot. Temporary fixation is obtained using cannulated pins and the position of the foot is checked with anteroposterior and lateral radiographs before definitive fixation with long, partially threaded cancellous screws. The wound is closed in layers and a large bulky dressing is applied, with a plaster splint incorporated into the bandage.

POSTOPERATIVE TREATMENT

Prophylactic intravenous antibiotics are used for 48 hours, the limb is elevated, and strict bed rest is enforced. Oral antibiotics are used until the wound is clean or the sutures are removed. Patients commence protected ambulation on the second postoperative day. No weight is allowed on the affected limb for 3 months and the foot is immobilized in a short leg cast. If patients are not able to comply with these restrictions after midfoot procedures, a rubber heel can be attached posteriorly on the cast to minimize pressure under the midfoot. Weightbearing is allowed when the warmth and swelling in the foot decrease, usually by 3 months. A reliable method of determining reduction of warmth is to use a skin thermistor and chart the changes in temperature every 2 to 3 weeks with the cast changes. The cast should be changed every 2 weeks during the first 6 weeks postsurgery and then at 3-week intervals. At approximately 3 months, weightbearing is commenced in a short leg cast for a further 3 months for the midfoot and for 6 to 12 additional months for the hindfoot and ankle. Once weightbearing has commenced, the foot should be inspected regularly. After midfoot procedures, patients should ambulate in a shoe with a rockerbottom sole and a protective molded orthosis should be provided and ready for the patient after casting is discontinued. The mold for the orthosis can be taken 4 weeks before the anticipated time for discontinuing the cast. A brace is not usually necessary for the midfoot, but is preferable for the hindfoot and ankle, where it is continued indefinitely.

SOFT-TISSUE RECONSTRUCTIVE SURGERY

With careful planning, the diabetic foot does lend itself to reconstructive procedures. The advent of microvascular surgery and deeper understanding of the vascular nature of diabetic degeneration have led to successful techniques for some previously untreatable problems.

A high rate of success with microvascular free-flap transfer has been demonstrated. Such grafts have been shown to provide coverage over large excised ulcer areas in the midfoot and hindfoot and that such transfers lead to marked improvement in the remaining foot secondary to increased tissue vascularity and improved regional oxygenation.

Such free-flap procedures rely on adequate macrovascular flow distally. If necessary, vascular bypass procedures can be performed initially in order to improve distal arterial flow. Using these techniques, the results following foot salvage can be dramatic, and with appropriate shoe wear modification, the patient can remain ambulatory.

The etiology of soft-tissue wounds in the diabetic patient is generally related to poor blood supply, neuropathy, pressure points from underlying bony deformity, and poor metabolic control of the underlying diabetic condition. Even if underlying skeletal deformity is corrected, the chronic severe bacterial colonization, osteomyelitis, severe wound fibrosis, and local wound ischemia make it very difficult for such

wounds to heal with simple debridement and dressing changes.

The historic notion that "small vessel disease" contributed to the diabetic wound resulted in a fatalistic view toward foot salvage in the diabetic patient. Recently, however, studies have failed to show any increased incidence of arteriolar disease in the diabetic patient, and have confirmed that ulceration may exist in the presence of normal transcutaneous oxygen tensions. This has pointed to accompanying peripheral neuropathy as the primary cause of foot wounds and has inspired new enthusiasm directed at getting these wounds to heal either with the use of local tissue or by microsurgical free tissue transfer.[82]

Infrapopliteal (tibioperoneal) vascular occlusion must be adequately evaluated so that prior to soft-tissue reconstruction, restoration of macrovascular blood flow is corrected by vascular bypass procedures. Evaluation of vascular status in the diabetic patient begins with a physical examination directed at identifying palpable dorsalis pedis and/or posterior tibial pulses, ruborous changes in the skin, suggestive of slowed circulatory transit time in the foot, as well as ulcers, fissures, and the presence or absence of hair growth. If strong pulses are not identified in at least one vessel in the foot, especially if there is ulceration present, vascular workup is indicated.

As has been recently noted, ankle-arm indices and Doppler noninvasive studies are fraught with error in the diabetic population because of the high incidence of vessel calcinosis, which leads to noncompressibility and, ultimately, a falsely elevated ankle pressure. Toe pressures, on the other hand, may be more helpful in light of the fact that the digital vessels are infrequently calcified. Pressures greater than 40 mm Hg generally reflect adequate local blood flow to allow wound healing. Colen[83] has popularized the use of directional Doppler studies, emphasizing that the normal Doppler blood flow velocity waveform is triphasic, consisting of forward flow, reverse flow, and a second forward flow component. Distal to an arterial stenosis or occlusion the waveform is dampened and the amplitude of wave velocity is decreased. As an arterial obstruction becomes more severe, the Doppler waveform actually deteriorates from triphasic to biphasic, and eventually from biphasic to monophasic to aphasic. Accordingly, patients with foot wounds and monophasic or aphasic waveforms should undergo vascular bypass surgery in order to restore macrovascular flow sufficient to sustain wound healing. Vascular bypass becomes essential if free tissue transfer is required for soft-tissue coverage to ensure adequate inflow of oxygenated blood into the free flap. Duplex Doppler imaging is also useful in order to identify recipient veins for vascular outflow. In the case of small wounds, amenable to coverage with local tissue, skin blood flow adequate to allow wound healing can be evaluated by $TCPO_2$. Generally, ulcers can heal if the $TCPO_2$ measurement exceeds 25 mm Hg.

Angiography is mandatory if either vascular surgical intervention or free flap reconstruction is necessary, as it provides anatomic information about vessel patency and size. In these cases, it is important to discuss the proposed angiogram with the radiologist and ensure that the study images the pedal arch in clear detail. Banis and associates[84] have emphasized that even in the absence of palpable pulses and angiographically visualized vessels, exploration and examination of distal vessels often results in a salvageable situation, noting that some perfusion of distal *viable* tissue must exist which implies that some vessels are open. Hence, high-grade proximal stenosis may prevent angiographic identification of distal vessels that are, in fact, patent. Although this may appear as an overly aggressive attempt to save a distal limb, there is great benefit in maintaining bipedal ambulation in a population whose risk for contralateral amputation is as high as 50% within 2 years.

The principles of wound management in a diabetic patient are no different than in the nondiabetic patient. Debridement of necrotic tissue and fibrotic wound edges must be complete. Underlying infected bone must be removed, and bony prominences must be addressed so that following soft-tissue restoration and wound healing, persistent pressure points do not contribute to recurrent breakdown.

The foot can be divided into four zones for the purpose of detailing reconstructive options (Fig. 25). These include the foot dorsum, the plantar forefoot, the weightbearing heel and midplantar area, and the posterior (nonweightbearing) heel, Achilles tendon, and malleoli. The reconstructive options for providing coverage for soft-tissue

FIGURE 25
Four zones of the foot. **1,** Posterior heel, Achilles tendon, and malleoli. **2,** Dorsum. **3,** Weightbearing heel and midplantar area. **4,** Plantar forefoot. (Courtesy of Lawrence B. Colen, MD, FACS, Norfolk, VA.)

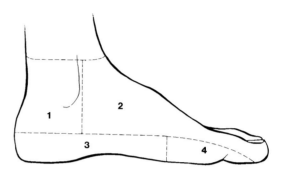

defects in each of these zones will be described below, however, it is important to remember certain fundamental principles critical to successful coverage. First, underlying bony prominence must be addressed. For example, if a metatarsophalangeal joint is subluxed or frankly dislocated, metatarsal head resection or metatarsal neck osteotomy should be performed at the time of wound closure. Similarly, if a patient has collapse of the midfoot with fixed deformity such that weightbearing is actually on the instep, resection of the prominence or, possibly, midfoot fusion should be considered at the time of soft-tissue coverage to prevent recurrent ulceration.

In each of these zones, local skin flaps or muscle transposition may effectively provide coverage. The caveat is that antegrade blood flow through the main feeding artery, whether it be the posterior tibial or anterior tibial, is essential. For the diabetic patient in whom peripheral vascular disease is widespread, local flaps are often unsuccessful because distal perfusion is inadequate. Thus, patients who have undergone recent distal vascular bypass procedures may not be suitable candidates for local arterialized flap coverage unless flow through these has been restored. In this situation, coverage may require the use of free tissue transfer. When distal vascular bypass surgery has been performed, direct arterial anastomosis to the bypass graft is always preferable (Figs. 26 through 32). If the revascularization has been performed proximally, it

FIGURE 26
Infected subtalar fusion on a 55-year-old diabetic man with peripheral vascular disease. (Courtesy of Lawrence B. Colen, MD, FACS, Norfolk, VA.)

FIGURE 27
Aphasic Doppler waveforms of the posterior tibial artery at the ankle. The waveform for the anterior tibia was no different. (Courtesy of Lawrence B. Colen, MD, FACS, Norfolk, VA.)

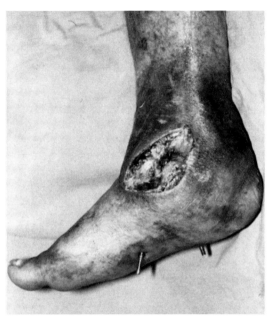

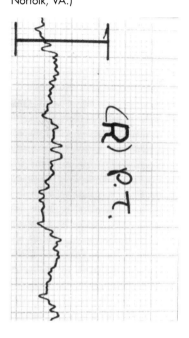

FIGURE 28
Left, The proximal portion of the saphenous vein bypass graft from the common femoral artery to the posterior tibial artery at the ankle. **Center,** The central portion of the vein bypass graft. **Right,** The distal portion of the graft at the ankle. (Courtesy of Lawrence B. Colen, MD, FACS, Norfolk, VA.)

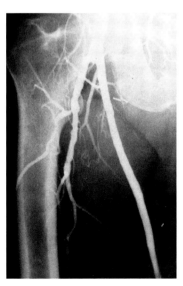 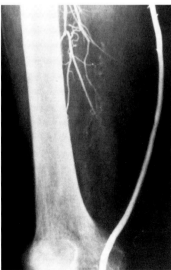 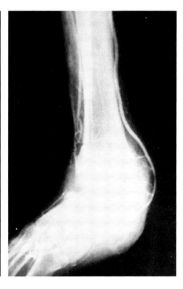

FIGURE 29
Almost biphasic Doppler waveform at the ankle following the bypass graft. (Courtesy of Lawrence B. Colen, MD, FACS, Norfolk, VA.)

FIGURE 30
Segment of the serratus anterior muscle, in situ, just prior to microvascular transfer. (Courtesy of Lawrence B. Colen, MD, FACS, Norfolk, VA.)

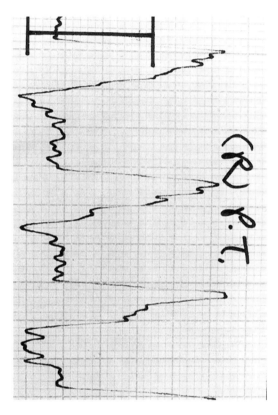

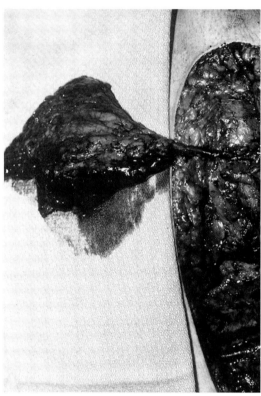

FIGURE 31
Diagrammatic representation of the procedure with anastomosis of the flap artery to the bypass graft at the ankle. (Courtesy of Lawrence B. Colen, MD, FACS, Norfolk, VA.)

FIGURE 32
Healing wound and successful fusion 3 years after surgery. (Courtesy of Lawrence B. Colen, MD, FACS, Norfolk, VA.)

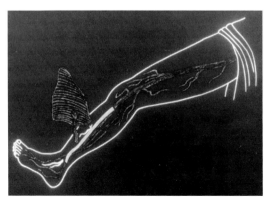

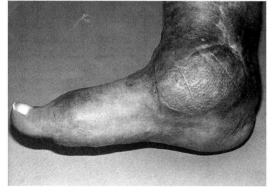

FIGURE 33
Infected Chopart's level amputation before (**top**) and after (**bottom**) debridement, and following latissimus muscle transfer. The patient currently bears weight without discomfort.

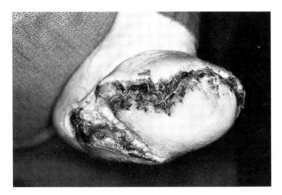
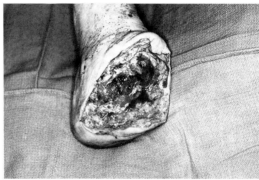
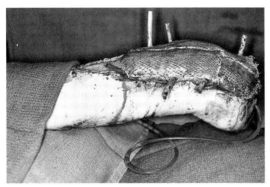
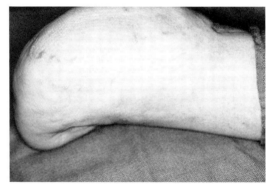

becomes critical to evaluate the suitability of the distal vasculature as recipient vessels for the transferred tissues.

FOOT DORSUM

Defects involving the dorsum of the foot are generally amenable to coverage with split thickness skin graft so long as a good base of granulation tissue can be achieved. If peritenon is lacking on the extensors, they may be excised without significant loss of foot function. If bone void of periosteum is exposed or a fibrotic devascularized base exists, skin grafting may not be successful and free tissue transfer may be required.

Ideally, a free flap would be thin and allow gliding beneath its surface to provide a favorable environment for subsequent tendon function. In practical terms, flap selection revolves around whether there is underlying infection of bone, because muscle flaps are superior to skin flaps in the presence of osteomyelitis. Most dorsal defects accompany wounds requiring transmetatarsal, Lisfranc, or Chopart level amputations, require free muscle flaps (rectus or latissimus) both in terms of their size, and the length and size of their pedicle (Fig. 33). In general, pedicles of upper limb flaps are relatively less involved with arterial sclerotic vascular disease than lower limb flaps, therefore, the gracilis is not often used in the diabetic patient. For smaller wounds requiring free tissue transfer, a serratus anterior free muscle flap is an excellent option.

PLANTAR FOREFOOT

The surgical treatment of forefoot wounds is based on their location. Obviously, isolated toe

FIGURE 34
Filet flap from toe for plantar forefoot
when following toe amputation.

FIGURE 35
V-Y advancement.

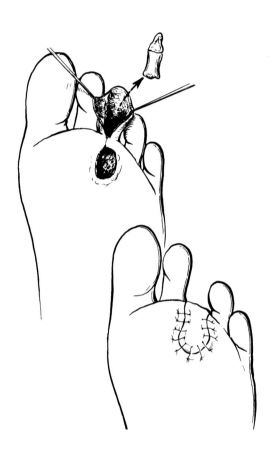

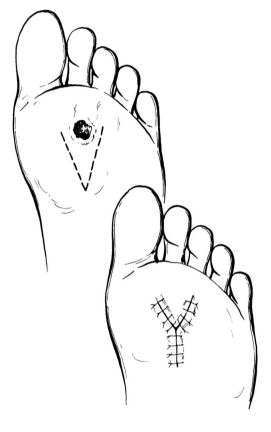

wounds can be treated by simple amputation so long as toe pressure and $TCPO_2$ measurements are compatible with healing.

Small ulcers underlying the metatarsal head can be addressed with "local" flaps using tissue from the toes or from the plantar aspect of the forefoot. If a toe requires amputation, filet of its soft-tissue envelope can often cover an ulcer of the metatarsal head (Fig. 34). Similarly, filet of an adjacent toe may provide enough tissue to close wounds 1 to 2 cm in size. The neurovascular island flap from the lateral side of the great toe, based either on the dorsal or plantar circulation, can be used to close defects approximating 2 to 3 cm. In this situation sacrifice of toe is not required, but antegrade distal flow is necessary

to supply the flap. Lastly, in light of a rich vascular supply to the plantar skin via perforators from the plantar artery through the fascia, V-Y advancement flaps provide an effective method of covering defects of 2 to 4 cm (Fig. 35).[85,86] Advancement of the flap is aided by careful but thorough division of all plantar fascia and most septal attachments, especially over the metatarsal heads.

When plantar ulceration involves the entire forefoot, transmetatarsal amputation may be a wiser option in terms of addressing the underlying bony cause of ulceration, and in these cases, free tissue transfer may be required for coverage (Fig. 36). The choices described above under reconstruction of dorsal defects remain applicable.

FIGURE 36
Rectus flap following transmetatarsal amputation.

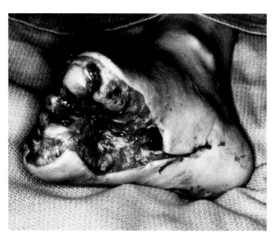

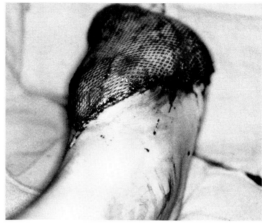

WEIGHTBEARING HEEL AND MIDPLANTAR AREA

Hildago and Shaw have provided a detailed list of potential local flaps that may provide coverage for small midplantar and weightbearing heel ulcers.[87] All but the lateral calcaneal artery flap require antegrade flow, and for that reason, are not always successful in a diabetic patient. The flexor digitorum brevis, abductor hallucis, and abductor digiti minimi muscles can be pedicled to reach the back of the heel without significant disruption of the plantar surface, but they are not recommended for coverage of defects over the malleoli.

The midplantar region of the foot may be elevated as a fasciocutaneous flap based on the medial plantar artery and transposed posteriorly to cover the heel. However, this requires skin grafting of the arch and as previously noted, is not a good choice in patients with midfoot collapse in whom the instep is a weightbearing unit.[88] Larger plantar hindfoot wounds (greater than 4 to 6 cm) or defects in patients without antegrade flow through the posterior tibial artery (which essentially supplies the three intrinsic foot muscles) must be reconstructed with microsurgical tissue transplantation. Currently, skin grafted muscle flaps are recommended because of their superior resistance to shear stresses, and their anticipated development of deep pressure sensation (Fig. 37). Innervated skin flaps are not recommended, especially in the diabetic population in whom sensory neuropathy is usually present.

POSTERIOR (NONWEIGHTBEARING) HEEL, ACHILLES TENDON, AND MALLEOLI

V-Y advancement flaps have been described for the reconstruction of skin defects of the posterior heel and ankle. Another useful option involves dissection of the extensor digitorum brevis muscle which can be used as a pedicled muscle flap based on the lateral tarsal artery and its source, the dorsalis pedis artery.[89] This muscle averages approximately 5 to 6 cm in size, and when completely isolated on the dorsalis pedis pedicle, provides coverage to either malleolus or the Achilles tendon area. As has been mentioned, however, its use requires antegrade flow through the anterior tibial and dorsalis pedis system. In the absence of infection, the thin coverage provided by a fasciocutaneous flap (radial forearm, lateral arm, scapular) is attractive (Fig. 38). In the presence of infection or fracture, however, muscle flap coverage is again advised because of superior blood supply and oxygen delivery compared to skin flaps.

FIGURE 37
Gracilis free flap for heel defect, before
(**left**) and after (**right**) transfer.

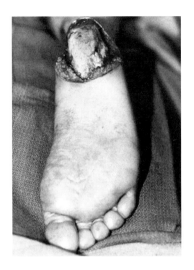
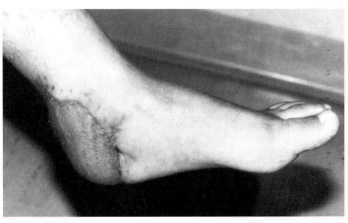

FIGURE 38
Photographs of free radial forearm flap
for medial heel defect before (**left**) and
after (**right**) transfer.

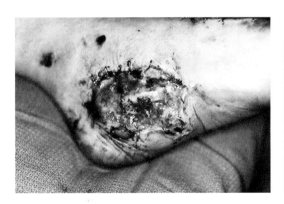
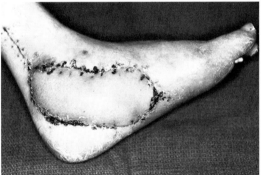

In summary, microsurgical techniques have been successfully applied to the patient with diabetes, but adequate macrovascular flow must exist. Coverage options, including skin grafting, local skin advancement, local muscle transposition, and free tissue transfer revolve around the location of the specific soft-tissue defect and the type of tissue required. In planning the reconstruction, the underlying bony framework must always be assessed and addressed, otherwise recurrent ulceration may develop. Postoperatively, adequate foot wear must be utilized in order to protect the reconstruction.

WOUND GROWTH FACTORS

Clinicians have long sought products to promote wound healing. Many specialized clinics devoted to wound care have noted success with resistant diabetic foot ulcer management. Although progress is often attributed to certain pharmaceuticals, much of the benefit is probably the result of a team approach to the problem. Constant patient and provider awareness and good wound management are the most important factors. Basic science research into wound healing has shown that as the wound begins to heal, platelet agglutination takes place as part of the blood clot formation that precedes fibroblastic ingrowth. The platelets release several "growth factors," among them, the platelet-derived growth factor (PDGF) and the more specific transforming growth factor beta (TGF-β). PDGF has an attraction for muscle cells and fibroblasts, and TGF-β demonstrates specific chemoattraction to inflammatory cells and fibroblasts. Both factors have been shown to be oxygen dependent.

Laboratory research has been impressive and early clinical studies have been favorable but not conclusive. At this time, no particular agent has universal acceptance.[82] There is no question that biologic enhancement to wound healing can be demonstrated; however, it seemingly is beneficial only as part of an organized and multidisciplinary approach to the total problem of the diabetic ulcer. Centers producing the best results from these agents are those that implement such technology as part of an overall treatment program.[90]

Among the more promising agents is CT-102, an activated platelet supernatant, which, in multicenter studies, has shown 80% wound healing versus placebo. The study by Steed and associates,[91] while quite promising, must be balanced with concerns over the safety of a blood-derived product.

As previously noted, diabetic foot ulcers can be "prevented" by reduction in the onset of neuropathy. Careful insulin management reduces the onset of neuropathic complications including foot ulcers. The usual twice-a-day insulin dosage is not as effective as more frequent dosing in maintaining relatively normal glucose levels.[92]

The acknowledged benefit of tighter insulin control has led to the development of insulin "pumps." These implanted devices can assist the patient in tailoring their insulin dosage to diet and activity fluctuations. While currently quite costly, their benefit may be shown to exceed current financial concerns when judged with respect to the cost of diabetic complications.

Among specific therapeutic agents designed to increase peripheral vascular function, pentoxifylline has shown some promise.[90] An 800 mg/day dosage was found to be effective in improving symptoms in noninsulin-dependent diabetics, and in nondiabetic patients a statistically significant improvement in ulcer healing was found. The case report would also suggest that it is beneficial with respect to the symptoms in both insulin and noninsulin-dependent diabetics. However, pentoxifylline's benefit in the treatment regimen of diabetic foot ulcers has as yet not been fully documented.

Pain in diabetic neuropathy can be severe and a challenging management problem. In an effort to find drugs other than narcotic pain medication, attention has turned to alternative biochemical approaches. Mexiletine, a sodium inhibitor with actions similar to those of lidocaine, has shown some improvement in pain relief in early reports.[93] Clonidine, an α-agonist, is also being used for pain control through its action on the sympathetic nervous system.[94] Both of these cardiovascular drugs have complex interactions and as yet limited clinical application.

HYPERBARIC OXYGEN

Tissue oxygenation at normal atmospheric pressure is maintained chiefly by the hemoglobin transport system of the red blood cells. However, the amount of oxygen available to tissues can be enhanced by increasing oxygen saturation in the plasma. A three-fold increase in plasma oxygenation is possible by the use of the hyperbaric oxygen chamber. Studies have demonstrated that this increase in oxygen-carrying capacity may persist beyond the time actually in the hyperbaric chamber. The increase in oxygen effect can be demonstrated for up to 6 hours after treatment.[16] The technique involves the

FIGURE 39
Hyperbaric oxygen. Large walk-in tank and smaller stretcher tank, Virginia Mason Hospital, Seattle, Washington.

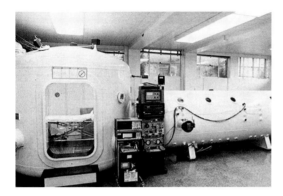

delivery of oxygen by a double seal mask or a hood to patients submitted to a 3 atm "dive" in a hyperbaric tank (Fig. 39). Such an increase is not possible through use of any regional or localized oxygen source, nor would the breathing of oxygen at a normal atmospheric pressure (sea level) be anticipated to result in such a prolonged oxygen increase.

The use of hyperbaric oxygen has been demonstrated to be beneficial in the treatment of soft-tissue clostridial infection, osteomyelitis, and compartment syndrome.[95,96] Application to the diabetic foot has been demonstrated to be effective[97] and relatively cost-effective,[98] in comparison to such efforts as outpatient intravenous antibiotics alone. Its use, however, remains somewhat tainted from past misapplications.

The decision to utilize hyperbaric oxygen should be predicated on the clinical determination that there is oxygen deprivation in the tissues and that enhanced delivery through the hyperbaric technique can be anticipated. Patients therefore must be screened for $TCPO_2$ levels. The patient's documented oxygen deficit should be improved by showing an adequate $TCPO_2$ response to 100% oxygen by mask at 1 atm. If an adequate response is not obtained and amputation is the only alternative, testing can be repeated in the hyperbaric chamber. If a significant rise in $TCPO_2$ occurs with either method, hyperbaric treatment is justified. Prior to treatment, the patient must also be screened for contraindications, such as significant cardiopulmonary disease, severe chronic obstructive pulmonary disease, or claustrophobia. The treatment program should be on a consistent basis, usually a minimum of five times per week, and of course be part of a continued general foot ulcer treatment protocol. A 70% success rate has been demonstrated in patients in whom all other treatment efforts had failed and for whom amputation remained the only alternative (Fig. 40).[99] The treatment technique consists of breathing mask 100% oxygen through a double seal mask or hood for three 30-minute sessions, separated by 10-minute breaks for a total of 90 minutes during a 2-hour "dive" to 2 to 4 atm. The number of treatments will be determined by the healing progress of the wound, but usually is a series of 20 to 30 treatments.

 CONCLUSION

The diabetic foot, like arteriosclerotic heart disease, cancer, and others of man's significant medical problems, does not yet have a simple "cure." Despite the lack of a cure, there has been great progress in treatment and prevention. The principles outlined in this publication have been shown to reduce the frequency of foot ulceration by half, to improve the time required to heal foot ulceration by two thirds, to reduce the amputation rate, and cut in half the mean length of inpatient treatment from 30 days to under 13 days.

To accomplish "the cure" with respect to diabetic foot ulcers is to make progress with prevention and to meticulously manage not only the foot ulcer but the patient's diabetic disease and its neurovascular complications. The orthopaedic surgeon and other health care professionals can make a difference by improving patient education and basic diabetic management, and by employing the current strategies in foot care management that have been outlined. No one modality, dressing, surgical procedure, or shoe wear modification is successful without the multidisciplinary and preferably the *team approach* to these complex problems.

FIGURE 40
Left, 39-year-old female after third toe amputation and femoropopliteal bypass.

Right, 30-month follow-up after 6 weeks of hyperbaric treatment.

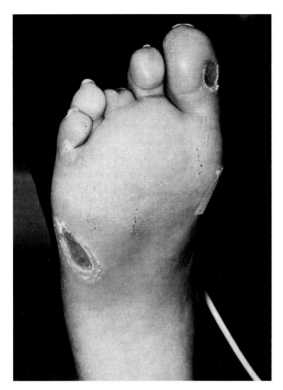

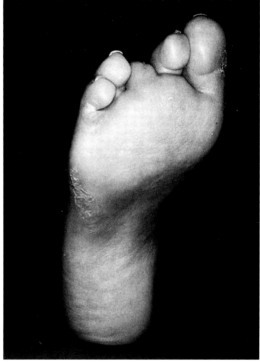

Diabetes is a complex problem. The challenge of management and the seriousness of potential complications necessitate an in-depth initial evaluation and a probing history. Patient noncompliance and the occult nature of progression make follow-up and ongoing Patient education an essential part of management.

The most universally accepted treatment of diabetic foot ulcers is to protect the ulcer in a tissue immobilized cast, where inflammatory response and ingrowth of granulation tissue can proceed undisturbed. Perhaps the most difficult ulcers to manage are those of the heel. Once established, the heel ulcer usually requires anatomic resection and a regional reconstruction. Successful treatment necessitates removal of all infected bone and of sufficient bone to allow easy skin closure without tension at the skin margins.

Diabetic foot infections are serious, often rapidly progressive conditions. Infections associated with neuropathic ulcers include cellulitis and abscess of the deep compartments of the foot. Foot infections are almost always caused by local invasion rather than hematogenous spread. Appropriate antibiotic selection covering aerobic and anaerobic organisms is important in managing the infection.

In amputations that result from diabetes or dysvascular foot problems, no well-defined criteria exist. The level of amputation is determined by functional considerations, the presence of infection, the status of the circulation, and the age and activity level of the patient. Local infection should not represent an impediment to amputation, but attention must be paid to the preoperative management of cellulitis and bacterial infection. Systemic sepsis is a relative contraindication and should be controlled prior to surgery, except in cases in which infection cannot be stabilized without the amputation of the infection site. The final decision with respect to amputation is based on predictability of healing. Although many types of testing are relatively successful, the level of $TCPO_2$ represents the best predictor of healing. In each case, the surgical procedure must be tailored to the limitations imposed by infection, deformity, and anticipated functions.

There are no absolute criteria regarding the use of postoperative antibiotics and they should be prescribed on an individual basis depending on the appearance of the wound. Intravenous antibiotics are recommended for approximately 10 days after surgery, followed by oral antibiotics as required.

The use of the total contact cast has immensely improved the postoperative management of these patients. It helps mobilize the patient rapidly, thereby avoiding many of the problems associated with prolonged bed rest. The presence of edema, local increases in temperature, and tenuous wound edges are all indications for continuing total contact cast treatment.

The Charcot foot is common in the diabetic patient and can ultimately lead to amputation of the limb. Although other elements of neuropathy and ischemia are often present, they may be addressed to some extent by revascularization without resorting to amputation. Structural breakdown of the foot (which leads to wound problems) and osteomyelitis are far more difficult to treat.

The goal of any treatment program for the Charcot foot is to achieve a plantigrade weight-bearing surface that is free of infection. In addition to these parameters, the foot and ankle must be stable and braceable. Whether the phase is acute or chronic and involves the midfoot, hindfoot, or ankle, most forms of Charcot breakdown are treated nonsurgically. The mainstay of treatment for neuropathic arthropathy, continues to be prolonged external immobilization in a plaster cast or brace. A brace is the traditional method of managing chronic deformity of the hindfoot and ankle. surgical treatment for neuropathic arthropathy of the foot and ankle is an option, but under most circumstances, this should not be the initial treatment of choice.

Ideally, surgery should not be performed in the presence of an open wound. Therefore, if feasible, wounds are first healed with either a total contact cast or a split-thickness skin graft. If surgery is performed in the presence of an open wound, the infection rate is increased. The treatment goal for patients with neuroarthropathy of the midfoot is to obtain a durable plantigrade foot for ambulation. To initiate appropriate treatment, it is important to identify the stage of neuroarthropathy. Once immobilization and rest bring active neuroarthropathy under control, a total contact cast becomes the mainstay of treatment.

The principles of wound management in a diabetic patient are no different than in the nondiabetic patient. Debridement of necrotic tissue and fibrotic wound edges must be complete. Underlying infected bone must be removed, and bony prominences must be addressed so that following soft-tissue restoration and wound healing, persistent pressure points do not contribute to recurrent breakdown.

Constant patient and provider awareness and good wound management are the most important factors in wound healing. PDGF and TGF-β have shown favorable but not conclusive results. Although biologic enhancement to wound healing can be demonstrated, it seemingly is beneficial only as part of an organized and multidisciplinary approach to the total problem of the diabetic ulcer.

The use of hyperbaric oxygen has been beneficial in the treatment of soft-tissue clostridial infection, osteomyelitis, and compartment syndrome. Application to the diabetic foot has been demonstrated to be effective and relatively cost-effective, in comparison to such efforts as outpatient intravenous antibiotics alone.

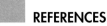

REFERENCES

1. Joslin EP: The universality of diabetes: A survey of diabetic morbidity in Arizona: Frank Billings lecture. *JAMA* 1940;115:2033-2038.

2. Sievers ML: Disease patterns among southwestern Indians. *Public Health Rep* 1966;81:1075-1083.

3. Sussman KE, Reiber G, Albert SF: The diabetic foot problem: A failed system of health care? *Diabetes Res Clin Pract* 1992;17:1-8.

4. Weinstein D, Wang A, Chambers R, et al: Evaluation of magnetic resonance imaging in the diagnosis of osteomyelitis in diabetic foot infections. *Foot Ankle* 1993;14:18-22.

5. Bodily KC, Burgess EM: Contralateral limb and patient survival after leg amputation. *Am J Surg* 1983;146:280-282.

6. Apelqvist J, Larsson J, Agardh CD: Long-term prognosis for diabetic patients with foot ulcers. *J Intern Med* 1993;233:485-491.

7. Aladin I: *Hong Kong.* Hong Kong, Government Information Services, 1989.

8. Ministry of Information: Singapore, 1991. Singapore, Publicity Promotions Divison, 1991.

9. Sugarman JR, Hickey M, Hall T, et al: The changing epidemiology of diabetes mellitus among Navajo Indians. *West J Med* 1990;153:140-145.

10. Das AK, Agarwal A: Letter. A precipitating factor in tropical diabetic foot ulcer in India. *J Assoc Physicians India* 1991;39:426.

11. Bondy PK: Disorders of carbohydrate metabolism: Diabetes mellitus, in Beeson PB, McDermott W (eds): *Textbook of Medicine,* ed 12. Philadelphia, PA, WB Saunders, 1967, pp 1175-1192.

12. Peakman M, Leslie RD, Vergani D: Immunological studies on type 1 diabetes in identical twins. *Arch Dis Child* 1993;69:97-99.

13. Fohlman J, Friman G: Is juvenile diabetes a viral disease? *Ann Med* 1993;25:569-574.

14. Flynn MD, Tooke JE: Aetiology of diabetic foot ulceration: A role for the microcirculation? *Diabet Med* 1992;9:320-329.

15. Vogelberg KH, Konig M: Hypoxia of diabetic feet with abnormal arterial blood flow. *Clin Investig* 1993;71:466-470.

16. McDermott JE: The diabetic foot: Evolving technologies, in Heckman JD (ed): *Instructional Course Lectures Volume 42.* Rosemont, IL, American Academy of Orthopaedic Surgeons, 1993, pp 169-171.

17. Barnett A: Prevention and treatment of the diabetic foot ulcer. *Br J Nursing* 1992;2:7-10.

18. Hickey H: Managing foot care cost. *Instride* 1993;6:3.

19. Reiber GE: Diabetic foot care: Financial implications and practice guidelines. *Diabetes Care* 1992;15:29-31.

20. Piaggesi A, Bini L, Castro Lopez E, et al: Knowledge on diabetes and performance among health professionals in non-diabetological departments. *Acta Diabetol* 1993;30:25-28.

21. Reenders K, de Nobel E, van den Hoogen HJ, et al: Diabetes and its long-term complications in general practice: A survey in a well-defined population. *Fam Pract* 1993;10:169-172.

22. McDermott JE: The diabetic foot: Diagnosis and prevention, in Heckman JD (ed): *Instructional Course Lectures Volume 42.* Rosemont, IL, American Academy of Orthopaedic Surgeons, 1993, pp 117-120.

23. Thompson C, McWilliams T, Scott D, et al: Importance of diabetic foot admissions at Middlemore Hospital. *N Z Med J* 1993;106:178-180.

24. Ewins DL, Bakker K, Young MJ, et al: Alternative medicine: Potential dangers for the diabetic foot. *Diabet Med* 1993;10:980-982.

25. Karanfilian RG, Lynch TG, Lee BC, et al: The assessment of skin blood flow in peripheral vascular disease by laser Doppler velocimetry. *Am Surg* 1984;50:641-644.

26. Karanfilian RG, Lynch TG, Zirul VT, et al: The value of laser Doppler velocimetry and transcutaneous oxygen tension determination in predicting healing of ischemic forefoot ulcerations and amputations in diabetic and nondiabetic patients. *J Vasc Surg* 1986;4:511-520.

27. Brodsky JW: Outpatient diagnosis and care of the diabetic foot, in Heckman JD (ed): *Instructional Course Lectures 42.* Rosemont, IL, American Academy of Orthopaedic Surgeons, 1993, pp 121-139.

28. McFadden JP, Corrall RJ, O'Brien IA: Autonomic and sensory nerve function in diabetic foot ulceration. *Clin Exp Dermatol* 1991;16:193-196.

29. Brodsky JW: The diabetic foot, in Mann RA, Coughlin MJ (eds): *Surgery of the Foot and Ankle,* ed 6. St. Louis, MO, Mosby Year Book, 1992, pp 1361-1467.

30. Wagner FW Jr: A classification and treatment program for diabetic, neuropathic, and dysvascular foot problems, in Cooper RR (ed): *American Academy of Orthopaedic Surgeons Instructional Course Lecture XXVIII.* St. Louis, MO, CV Mosby, 1979, pp 143-165.

31. Wagner FW Jr: The diabetic foot. *Orthopedics* 1987;10:163-172.

32. Steed DL, Goslen JB, Holloway GA, et al: Randomized prospective double-blind trial in healing chronic diabetic foot ulcers: CT-102 activated platelet supernatant, topical versus placebo. *Diabetes Care* 1992;15:1598-1604.

33. Chantelau E, Breuer U, Leisch AC, et al: Outpatient treatment of unilateral diabetic foot ulcers with "half shoes." *Diabet Med* 1993;10:267-270.

34. Brodsky JW, Kourosh S, Stills M, et al: Objective evaluation of insert material for diabetic and athletic footwear. *Foot Ankle* 1988;9:111-116.

35. Myerson M, Wilson K: Management of neuropathic ulceration with the total contact cast, in Sammarco GJ (ed): *The Foot in Diabetes*. Philadelphia, PA, Lea & Febiger, 1991, pp 145-152.

36. Myerson M, Papa J, Eaton K, et al: The total-contact cast for management of neuropathic plantar ulceration of the foot. *J Bone Joint Surg* 1992;74A:261-269.

37. Helm PA, Walker SC, Pullium G: Total contact casting in diabetic patients with neuropathic foot ulcerations. *Arch Phys Med Rehabil* 1984;65:691-693.

38. Smith WJ, Jacobs RL, Fuchs MD: Salvage of the diabetic foot with exposed os calcis. *Clin Orthop* 1993;296:71-77.

39. Gentry LO: Diagnosis and management of the diabetic foot ulcer. *J Antimicrob Chemother* 1993;32(suppl A):77-89.

40. Pratt TC: Gangrene and infection in the diabetic. *Med Clin North Am* 1965;49:987-1004.

41. Delbridge L, Ctercteko G, Fowler C, et al: The aetiology of diabetic neuropathic ulceration of the foot. *Br J Surg* 1985;72:1-6.

42. Savin JA: Bacterial infections in diabetes mellitus. *Br J Dermatol* 1974;91:481-484.

43. Brisco HF, Allison F Jr: Diabetes and host resistance: I. Effect of alloxan diabetes upon the phagocytic and bactericidal efficiency of rat leukocytes for *Pneumococcus. J Bacteriol* 1965;90:1537-1541.

44. Dolkart RE, Halpern B, Perlman J: Comparison of antibody responses in normal and alloxan diabetic mice. *Diabetes* 1971;20:162-167.

45. Kass EH: Hormones and host resistance to infection. *Bacteriol Rev* 1960;24:177-185.

46. Marble A, White HJ, Fernald AT: The nature of the lowered resistance to infection in diabetes mellitus. *J Clin Invest* 1938;17:423-430.

47. Wale RS, Madders K: Staphylococcal toxoid in the treatment of diabetes. *Br J Exp Pathol* 1936;17:279-281.

48. Brayton RG, Stokes PE, Schwartz MS, et al: Effect of alcohol and various diseases on leukocyte mobilization, phagocytosis, and intracellular bacterial killing. *N Engl J Med* 1970;282:123-128.

49. Dziatkowiak H, Kowalska M, Denys A: Phagocytic and bactericidal activity of granulocytes in diabetic children. *Diabetes* 1982;31:1041-1043.

50. Fortes ZB, Farsky SP, Oliveira MA, et al: Direct vital microscopic study of defective leukocyte-endothelial interaction in diabetes mellitus. *Diabetes* 1991;40:1267-1273.

51. Nolan CM, Beaty HN, Bagdade JD: Further characterization of the impaired bactericidal function of granulocytes in patients with poorly controlled diabetes. *Diabetes* 1978;27:889-894.

52. Perillie PE, Nolan JP, Finch SC: Studies of the resistance to infection in diabetes mellitus: Local exudative cellular response. *J Lab Clin Med* 1962;59:1008-1015.

53. Sima AA, O'Neill SJ, Naimark D, et al: Bacterial phagocytosis and intracellular killing by alveolar macrophages in BB rats. *Diabetes* 1988;37:544-549.

54. Tan JS, Anderson JL, Watanakunakorn C, et al: Neutrophil dysfunction in diabetes mellitus. *J Lab Clin Med* 1975;85:26-33.

55. Tachibana DK: Microbiology of the foot. *Annu Rev Microbiol* 1976;30:351-375.

56. Newrick PG, O'Brien IA, Smart A, et al: Impaired sweating in the diabetic neuropathic foot and its influence on skin flora. *Diabetes Res* 1989;12:173-176.

57. Leichter SB, Allweiss P, Harley J, et al: Clinical characteristics of diabetic patients with serious pedal infections. *Metab Clin Exper* 1988;37(2 Suppl 1):22-24.

58. Kozak GP, Rowbotham JL: Diabetic foot disease: A major problem, in Kozak GP, Hoar CS Jr, Rowbotham JL, et al (eds): *Management of Diabetic Foot Problems: Joslin Clinic and New England Deaconess Hospital*. Philadelphia, PA, WB Saunders, 1984, pp 1-8.

59. Newman LG, Waller J, Palestro CJ, et al: Comments. Unsuspected osteomyelitis in diabetic foot ulcers: Diagnosis and monitoring by leukocyte scanning with indium In 111 oxyquinoline. *JAMA* 1992;267:510-511.

60. Levin S: Digest of current literature. *Infect Dis Clin Prac* 1992;1:49-50.

61. Bessman AN, Geiger PJ, Canawati H: Prevalence of *Corynebacteria* in diabetic foot infections. *Diabetes Care* 1992;15:1531-1533.

62. Wang A, Weinstein D, Greenfield L, et al: MRI and diabetic foot infections. *Magn Reson Imaging* 1990;8:805-809.

63. Lipsky BA, Pecoraro RE, Larson SA, et al: Outpatient management of uncomplicated lower-extremity infections in diabetic patients. *Arch Intern Med* 1990;150:790-797.

64. Drachman RH, Root RK, Wood WB Jr: Studies on the effect of experimental nonketotic diabetes mellitus on antibacterial defense: I. Demonstration of a defect in phagocytosis. *J Exp Med* 1966;124:227-240.

65. Parkhouse N, Le Quesne PM: Impaired neurogenic vascular response in patients with diabetes and neuropathic foot lesions. *N Engl J Med* 1988;318:1306-1309.

66. Criado E, De Stefano AA, Keagy BA, et al: The course of severe foot infection in patients with diabetes. *Surg Gynecol Obstet* 1992;175:135-140.

67. Tannenbaum GA, Pomposelli FB Jr, Marcaccio EJ, et al: Safety of vein bypass grafting to the dorsal pedal artery in diabetic patients with foot infections. *J Vasc Surg* 1992;15:982-990.

68. Pinzur MS: Amputation level selection in the diabetic foot. *Clin Orthop* 1993;296:68-70.

69. Myerson MS, Bowker JH, Brodsky JW, et al: Symposium: Partial foot amputations. *Contemp Orthop* 1994;29:139-157.

70. Jacobs RL: Salvage of a functional lower limb in diabetic patients after amputation, in Heckman JD (ed): *Instructional Course Lectures 42*. Rosemont, IL, American Academy of Orthopaedic Surgeons, 1993, pp 159-167.

71. Due TM, Jacobs RL: Molded foot orthosis after great toe or medial ray amputations in diabetic feet. *Foot Ankle* 1985;6:150-152.

72. Gupta R: A short history of neuropathic arthropathy. *Clin Orthop* 1993;296:43-49.

73. Eichenholtz SN: *Charcot Joints*. Springfield, IL, Charles C. Thomas, 1966.

74. Myerson M, Alvarez RG, Brodsky JW, et al: Symposium: Neuroarthropathy of the foot. *Contemp Orthop* 1993;26:43-64.

75. Saltzman CL, Johnson KA, Goldstein RH, et al: Patella tendon bearing brace as treatment for neurotrophic arthropathy: A diabetic force monitoring study. *Foot Ankle* 1992;13:14-21.

76. Papa J, Myerson M, Girard P: Salvage, with arthrodesis, in intractable diabetic neuropathic arthropathy of the foot and ankle. *J Bone Joint Surg* 1993;75A:1056-1066.

77. Myerson M: Arthrodesis for diabetic neuroarthropathy, in Myerson M (ed): *Current Therapy in Foot and Ankle Surgery*. St. Louis, MO, Mosby Year Book, 1993, pp 116-122.

78. Shibata T, Tada K, Hashizume C: The results of arthrodesis of the ankle for leprotic neuroarthropathy. *J Bone Joint Surg* 1990;72A:749-756.

79. Stuart MJ, Morrey BF: Arthrodesis of the diabetic neuropathic ankle joint. *Clin Orthop* 1990;253:209-211.

80. Myerson MS, Henderson MR, Saxby T, et al: Management of midfoot diabetic neuroarthropathy. *Foot Ankle Int* 1994;15:233-241.

81. Sinha S, Munichoodappa CS, Kozak GP: Neuroarthropathy (Charcot joints) in diabetes mellitus (clinical study of 101 cases). *Medicine* 1972;51:191-210.

82. Lo Gerfo FW, Gibbons GW, Pomposelli FB Jr, et al: Trends in the care of the diabetic foot: Expanded role of arterial reconstruction. *Arch Surg* 1992;127:617-621.

83. Colen LB: Limb salvage in the patient with severe peripheral vascular disease: The role of microsurgical free-tissue transfer. *Plast Reconstr Surg* 1987;79:389-395.

84. Banis JC Jr, Richardson JD, Derr JW, et al: Microsurgical adjuncts in salvage of the ischemic and diabetic lower extremity. *Clin Plast Surg* 1992;19:881-893.

85. Maruyama Y, Iwahira Y, Ebilhara H: V-Y advancement flaps in the reconstruction of skin defects of the posterior heel and ankle. *Plast Reconstr Surg* 1990;85:759-764.

86. Colen LB, Replogle SL, Mathes SI: The V-Y plantar flap for reconstruction of the forefoot. *Plast Reconstr Surg* 1988;81:220-228.

87. Hildago DA, Shaw WW: Reconstruction of foot injuries. *Clin Plast Surg* 1986;13:663-680.

88. Shaw WW, Hidalgo PA: Anatomic basis of plantar foot design. *Clin Applications* 1986;78:637-649.

89. Giordano PA, Argenson C, Pequignot JP: Extensor digitorum brevis as an island flap in the reconstruction of soft-tissue defects in the lower limb. *Plast Reconstr Surg* 1989;83:100-109.

90. Campbell RK: Clinical update on pentoxifylline therapy for diabetes-induced peripheral vascular disease. *Ann Pharmacother* 1993;27:1099-1105.

91. Steed DL, Goslen JB, Holloway GA, et al: Randomized prospective double-blind trial in healing chronic diabetic foot ulcers: CT-102 activated platelet supernatant, topical versus placebo. *Diabetes Care* 1992;15:1598-1604.

92. Grunfeld C: Diabetic foot ulcers: Etiology, treatment, and prevention. *Adv Intern Med* 1992;37:103-132.

93. Stracke H, Meyer UE, Schumacker HE: Mexiletine in the treatment of diabetic neuropathy. *Diabetes Care* 1992;15:1550-1555.

94. Belgrade MJ, Lev BI: Diabetic neuropathy: Helping patients cope with this pain. *Postgrad Med* 1991;90:263-270.

95. Esterhai JL, Pisarello J, Brighton CT, et al: Treatment of chronic refractory osteomyelitis with adjunctive hyperbaric oxygen. *Orthop Rev* 1988;17:809-815.

96. Strauss MB, Hart GB: Hyperbaric oxygen and the skeletal muscle-compartment syndrome. *Contemp Orthop* 1989;18:167.

97. Doctor N, Pandya S, Supe A: Hyperbaric oxygen therapy in the diabetic foot. *J Postgrad Med* 1992;38:112-114.

98. Ciani P, Petrone G, Drager S: Salvage of the problem wound and potential amputation with wound care and adjunctive hyperbaric oxygen therapy: An economic analysis. *J Hyperbaric Med* 1989;3:127.

99. Griffiths GD, Wieman TJ: Meticulous attention to foot care improves the prognosis in diabetic ulceration of the foot. *Surg Gynecol Obstet* 1992;174:49-51.

INDEX

Page numbers in italics refer to figures or figure legends.